Kettlebells

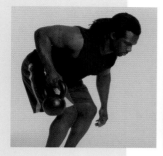
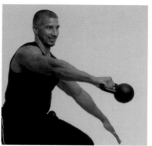

Kettlebells

Strength Training for Power & Grace

Smith Vatel, BS, CSCS, and Victoria D. Gray, MPA, ATC

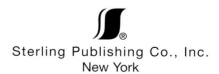
Sterling Publishing Co., Inc.
New York

Library of Congress Cataloging-in-Publication Data Available

2   4   6   8   10   9   7   5   3   1

Published by Sterling Publishing Co., Inc.
387 Park Avenue South, New York, NY 10016
Copyright © 2005 by Smith Vatel and Victoria D. Gray
Distributed in Canada by Sterling Publishing
c/o Canadian Manda Group, 165 Dufferin Street
Toronto, Ontario, Canada M6K 3H6
Distributed in the United Kingdom by GMC Distribution Services,
Castle Place, 166 High Street, Lewes, East Sussex, England BN71XU
Distributed in Australia by Capricorn Link (Australia) Pty Ltd.
P.O. Box 704, Windsor, NSW 2756, Australia

For information about custom editions, special sales, premium and
corporate purchases, please contact Sterling Special Sales
Department at 800-805-5489 or specialsales@sterlingpub.com.

Sterling ISBN 13: 978-1-4027-2758-0
ISBN 10: 1-4027-2758-5

contents

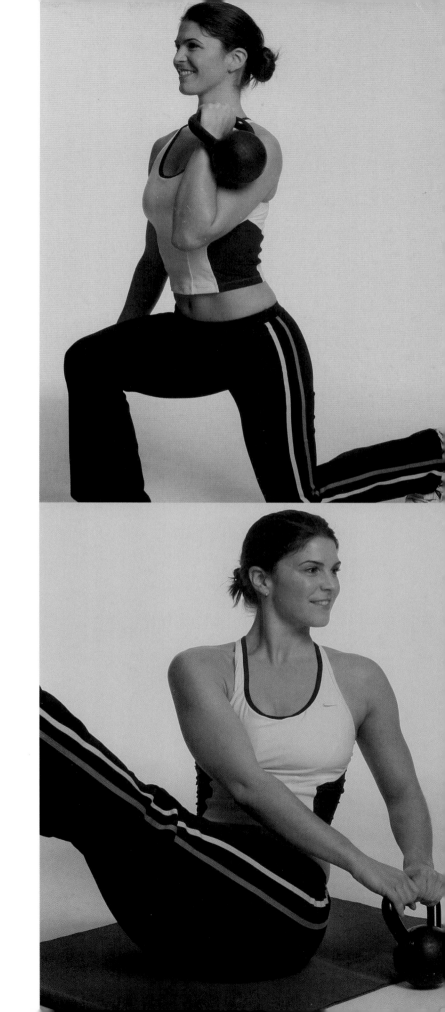

introduction

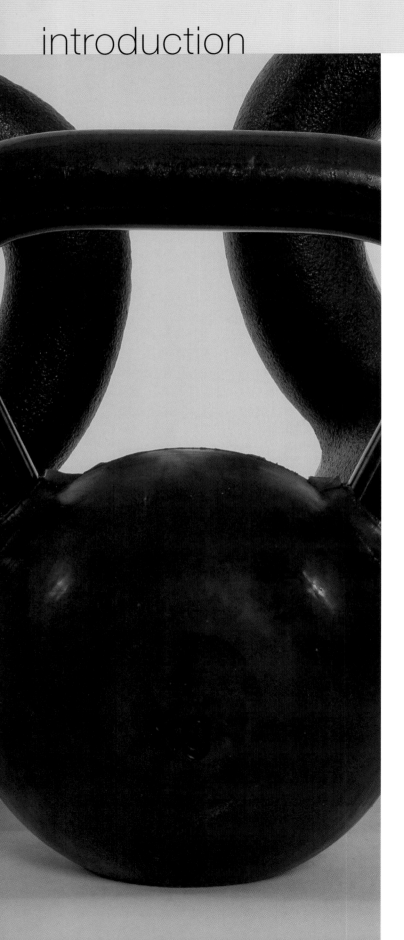

INTRODUCING KETTLEBELLS

A cast iron kettlebell, commonly known as a *girya* in Russia, looks like a cannonball with a handle. Unlike other forms of weight lifting, training with a kettlebell uses momentum along with gravity to train the entire body as a unit. In addition, the fluid motion improves joint flexibility. By swinging the kettlebell and keeping it in motion, you train for strength and cardiovascular endurance at the same time. And, because kettlebell exercises use large muscle movements, you burn a tremendous number of calories in every session, providing you with a quick way to increase lean muscle mass, lose fat, and gain endurance and flexibility. Mastering the art of kettlebells is challenging, but practiced over time, you'll see tremendous fitness gains.

It's not surprising that kettlebells have recently become popular again and are being used by fitness enthusiasts, professional athletes, martial artists, the U.S. military, and law enforcement officers. Although kettlebells have been around for more than a century in Eastern Europe, nobody really knows exactly when or how they evolved. Legend has it that they have been used for years by Russian strongmen, athletes, and the Spetsnaz (Soviet Special Forces). At one point, exercising with kettlebells was so popular in Russia that it was considered a national sport.

Over the last fifty years, dumbbells and plate-loaded barbells have largely displaced kettlebells from gyms, and the knowledge of how to use them has disappeared as well. The difficult part about working with kettlebells is that, although the equipment is exceedingly simple, kettlebells require certain basic skills and techniques before you can master their use. This book can help you master the proper posture, grips, pacing, and movements. It also provides dozens of exercises that you can add to your training routine. You'll learn how to adapt dumbbell or barbell movements (such as dead lifts and squats) to train with kettlebells; how to train your body to deal with the absorption of forces by accelerating and decelerating weight properly; and how to design effective full-body workouts that match your goals and conditioning needs.

Performed with a lighter weight and more repetitions, kettlebell exercises also build up your muscular endurance. Muscle endurance training enhances your ability to continue lifting weight over an extended period of time while increasing your resistance to fatigue. Strength training will also have a positive effect on your body's composition. Greater muscle mass will burn more calories, reduce fat tissue, and increase your metabolic rate, helping you to accomplish your weight loss and overall wellness goals.

THE BALANCED WORKOUT

A well-rounded fitness regime includes cardiovascular endurance training, muscular strength and endurance training, and flexibility training. How can you get a cardiovascular, muscle strength, muscle endurance and flexibility training program and still be efficient with your time? The answer to this question is kettlebells.

Muscular strength training should aim to improve both muscular strength (how much weight you can lift) and muscular endurance (how many times or how long you can lift a weight). Most of your muscles have two types of fibers: fast-twitch muscle fibers (type II fibers), which can be trained to provide explosive force, and slow-twitch fibers (type I fibers), which can be trained to reduce fatigue in endurance exercises. Quick movements engage your fast-twitch muscle fibers, while sustained efforts rely on slow-twitch muscle fibers. Kettlebell exercises performed with heavy weight (a weight that can be lifted with proper form for ten repetitions or less) primarily build muscular strength, while exercises performed with a lighter weight and more repetitions build muscular endurance. You should incorporate both types of training into your routine.

Kettlebell workouts can provide a cardiovascular workout as well. Once you're adept at kettlebell motion and you're able to apply continuous, vigorous motion in your workout, your heart rate will stay high, providing an excellent cardiovascular workout. Cardiovascular training should be a major part of your fitness program because it increases your capacity to use oxygen while it conditions your heart, decreasing your risk of heart disease, stroke, and high blood pressure. Complement your cardiovascular training with other continuous motion activities such as running, biking, or aerobic classes on alternate days.

Finally, kettlebells are excellent for flexibility training, which helps you achieve a greater range of motion in your joints. The momentum of the kettlebell exercises encourages a full range of motion, which stimulates the synovial fluid that allows your joints to move smoothly. These fluid movements will increase your joint flexibility over time and can help to reduce the effects of arthritis, as well as providing you with a sense of grace in motion. You'll get extra benefits if you complement kettlebell training with stretching, yoga, or even a dance class. Flexibility training should be done after you have warmed up your muscle fibers with a few minutes of aerobic activity. Although you may not see the same immediate or dramatic results with flexibility training as you would doing a cardiovascular or strength-training program, participating in a regular flexibility training program several times a week will help you maintain your body's mobility and range of movement. Additionally, a flexibility training program can be an integral part of a rehabilitation or injury prevention program if tight muscle groups are a contributing factor. Above all, incorporating a flexibility training program into your fitness regime will help you relax, both physically and mentally.

How do you add kettlebells to your fitness regimen? You should consider kettlebells another technique for improving your fitness. They provide an excellent supplement to your routine when you are focusing on improving power and speed. A kettlebell workout is always a great choice when you are pressed for time because you work out your whole body, and if you keep moving, it counts as a cardiovascular workout as well as a weight-lifting session. As with any workout regime, you should continually change your routine to challenge your body. Alternate your kettlebell routine with all the other exercise disciplines you enjoy, such as traditional strength training, yoga, running, biking, boxing, and/or group fitness classes. You should always give yourself forty-eight hours of rest between kettlebell sessions to avoid overtraining and to reduce the potential for injury, especially because it is difficult to isolate different body parts in training. Remember to change the specific exercises within each workout session at least every two weeks. See the sample routines on pages 120–125 for ideas about how to put together your workout. This will keep you on course for obtaining your fitness goals.

getting started

EQUIPMENT

The weight of Russian kettlebells is measured in poods. One pood is approximately 35 pounds (16 kilograms). Traditionally, kettlebells came in three different sizes: one pood, one and a half poods, and two poods. Today, you can find kettlebells in many different sizes, starting as small as 9 pounds (4 kilograms, or .25 poods) and going all the way up to 88 pounds (40 kilograms, or 2.5 poods).

Before purchasing a kettlebell for your workout routine, you should consider whether you would like a traditional cast iron kettlebell, adjustable kettlebells (stackable plates that are color-coded to help you set your desired weight), vinyl iron kettlebells, or new-on-the-scene colored kettlebells. Below are are the weight conversions from poods to approximate pounds and kilograms:

.25 poods	—	approx. 9 lbs (4 kg)
.50 poods	—	approx. 18 lbs (8 kg)
.75 poods	—	approx. 26 lbs (12 kg)
1 pood	—	approx. 35 lbs (16 kg)
1.25 poods	—	approx. 44 lbs (20 kg)
1.5 poods	—	approx. 53 lbs (24 kg)
1.75 poods	—	approx. 62 lbs (28 kg)
2 poods	—	approx. 70 lbs (32 kg)
2.5 poods	—	approx. 88 lbs (40 kg)

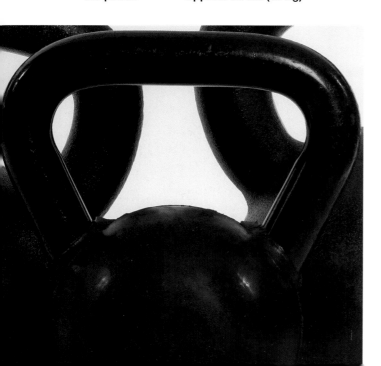

How to Choose the Correct Weight

An average man should start with the 1 pood (35 lbs/16 kg) kettlebell. Most fit women should start with the .50 pood (18 lbs/8 kg) kettlebell. If you are new to strength training, you should choose one of the lighter weights. You should progress in weight once you have become acccomplished with the kettlebell movements. Remember, due to the complex nature of a kettlebell routine and the use of momentum, you will not be able initially to lift the amount of weight as you might expect. Do not expect your kettlebell weight to be the same weight you can lift in a bench press, especially when performing the more challenging combination exercises.

Where to Find Kettlebells

At this writing, kettlebells aren't widely available for purchase at many retailers, but you can order them direct from manufacturers. (See page 126 to choose from the many Web sites where kettlebells are available.)

How to Make Your Own Kettlebell

Kettlebells may be pricey and hard to find, but there are alternatives: You may use regular dumbbells to perform kettlebell movements, although this will not be as effective, as it will not challenge your balance in the same way (a kettlebell is special because its weight is concentrated in the middle, not on either side). A better alternative is to use household products to create a less expensive version. One option is to fill a plastic gallon jug with sand, salt, gravel, or even water. Test your jug for cracks and leaks before beginning your routine. To get the right balance, you must have the weight in the center, which gives you the ability to swing the weight.

Nonetheless, we recommend that you make the investment and purchase an original cast iron kettlebell. You will be better able to perform the movements and advance yourself accordingly with the proper equipment—and it still costs much less than a full set of traditional weights.

Setting Up Your Workout Space

You do not need a huge space, which is why kettlebells are ideal for a home workout. If you are starting a kettlebell routine in your home, you will need a clear space that is free of all

WARNING: Consider your surroundings. If you are planning on starting a kettlebell routine at home and you have breakable objects around, or your space is tight, the best place to perform your kettlebell routine is outside.

objects—including pets and other people! You will need enough space to swing the kettlebell forward to shoulder level without hitting anything. You should be able to stand in your room with your feet slightly wider than shoulder width and to extend your arms out to the side without touching any objects (approximately 14 to 16 square feet).

SAFETY PRECAUTIONS

- Be aware of your surroundings and keep them clear of objects. Choose an area that has a sturdy, nonslip floor. Yoga or wrestling mats work well.
- Allow for sufficient rest, at least 48 hours between each kettlebell workout, to prevent overtraining and potential injury.
- Take time to understand each exercise before starting your workout. Remember, unlike lifting stationary weights, momentum is critical with kettlebells.
- Store your kettlebell out of reach of children and anyone who might use them incorrectly.
- You should be free of distractions when starting your kettlebell routine. It is very dangerous to be working with your kettlebells and to have a pet or family member run into the room. Small children can make unexpected movements, get in your way while you're working with weights, and be injured.
- Be sure to wear appropriate workout clothes (nothing too baggy) and sneakers or athletic shoes that have soles with good grips. Running shoes are not suggested because they do not support the foot well when performing lateral movement. We recommend wearing cross-trainers.
- Before starting any exercise program, you should consult your physician. If you are pregnant, have or have had previous injuries that could be made worse with physical activity, or have a heart condition, you need to see your doctor before starting this or any kettlebell/exercise regime.

POSTURE

Good posture is critical for any workout program, but because kettlebells require the use of momentum with movement, it is easy to lose correct posture. Focus on maintaining correct posture all the way through the movement to prevent injuries. Correct posture will also improve your results by helping you learn to absorb outside forces, and will increase the effectiveness of each movement by engaging the abdominal and pelvic stabilizing muscles.

Correct Posture
- Stand with your head up and your neck long and straight
- Look straight ahead
- Pull your shoulders back
- Relax your arms by your side
- Engage your abdominal muscles
- Hold your pelvis with a slight posterior tilt
- Bend your knees slightly
- Keep your legs hip-width apart
- Keep your feet flat on the floor and pointed forward

Incorrect Posture
- Head flexed forward, looking down at the ground
- Shoulders rounded forward
- Back rounded
- Abdominal muscles loose
- Knees locked
- Legs loose
- Neck arched

WARMING UP

It is very important to make sure that all your muscles have a good supply of blood and oxygen before starting your workout program. Because of the use of momentum with kettlebells, it is critical to focus on a total body warm-up, which can be done by running in place, doing jumping jacks, jumping rope, or doing arm circles (clockwise and counterclockwise) or using the kettlebell double-arm swing squat exercise (see pages 20–21). Your warm-up should take about five to ten minutes.

Now that your muscles have oxygen and a good supply of blood, you should perform a couple of stretches before starting your kettlebell routine. To help increase the range of motion in your joints (critical to avoiding injury while performing your kettlebell routine), focus on stretching your calves, hamstrings, quadriceps, hip flexors, glutes, chest, shoulders, and triceps. Also remember to stretch your lateral, diagonal, and forward neck flexors.

ANATOMY

The illustrations below will help you visualize the major muscle groups activated during a kettlebell routine.

REPS, SETS, AND TEMPO

Repetition maximum (RM) is the maximum number of times you can lift the kettlebell according to its load (weight). Many fitness professionals speak of a one-repetition maximum, which is the amount of weight an individual can lift at one time. A set is a predetermined number of repetitions (reps). Keep in mind that your sets and reps will vary according to your fitness goals, age, sex, physical condition, and health. Always remember that what may seem heavy to you may or may not be heavy for someone else.

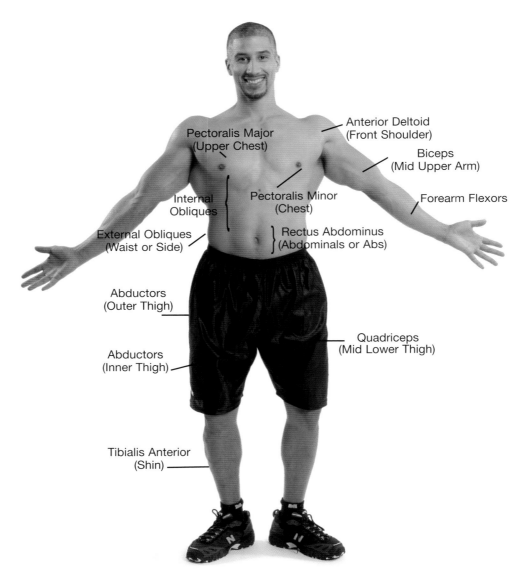

Anterior Muscles

Tempo refers to the pace at which you perform the kettlebell movements, from start to finish. Whenever you are working with kettlebells, you should pick a tempo that allows you to execute the movement as fast as possible without compromising your form. The tempos we have suggested in this book should be used only as a guideline. Initially, you may choose a slower tempo, but as you perfect the movements you will be able to increase your speed.

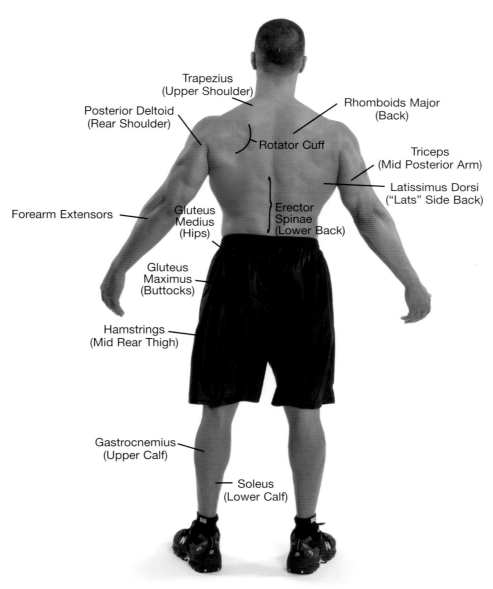

Posterior Muscles

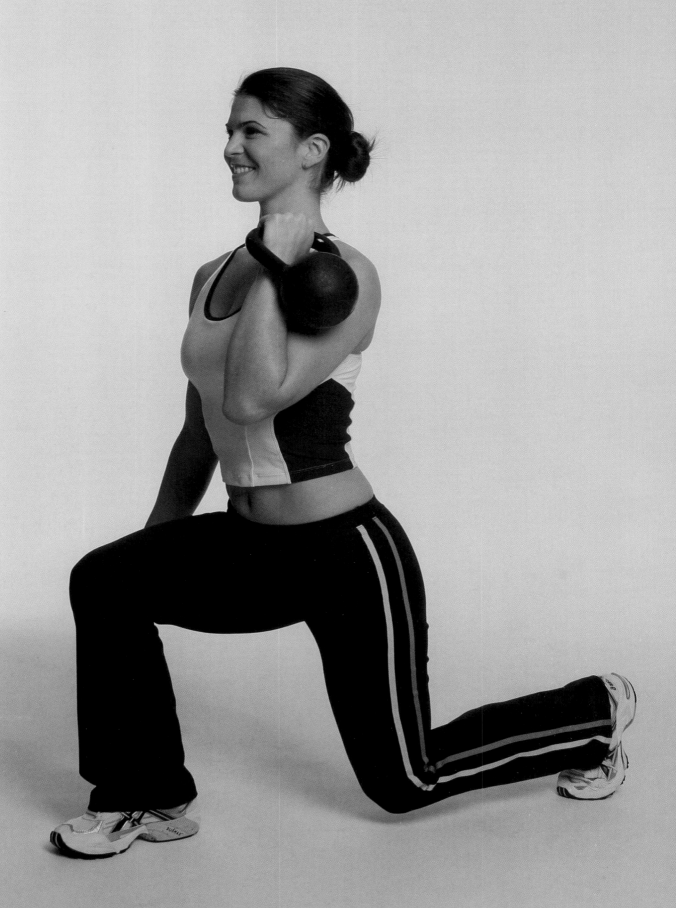

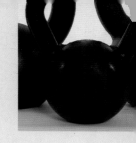

the essential moves

kettlebell grip positions

There are three different grip positions for the kettlebell exercises illustrated in this book. Initially, you should start with the *rack grip position*. This position is the most stable of the three, as it requires less balance while performing coordinated and momentum exercises. Once you feel comfortable and can perform the exercises with a fluid motion, you should progress to the *waiter grip position*, which is less stable than the rack and will challenge your ability to stabilize the kettlebell during the exercises. Again, you should progress only when you can perform the combination and momentum exercises with a fluid and graceful motion. The third grip is the *bottoms-up grip position*, which requires greater joint stability and ability to balance the kettlebell throughout the exercise. When trying the different grip positions, you should progress as suggested, only when you are ready, to limit your risk of injury. The bottoms-up grip is the most challenging of the three and naturally poses greater risk.

These illustrations will give you a closer look at the individual grip positions.

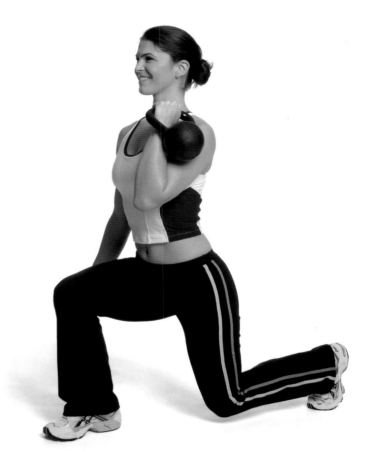

Rack Position

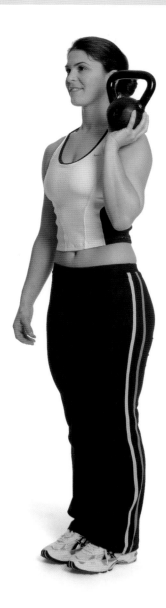

Waiter Position

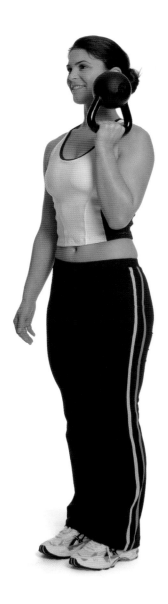

Bottoms-up Position

kettlebell squat

The squat is an essential movement of daily life. The squat is most often used when lowering yourself to sit in a chair and returning to a standing position. It is also the basis of nearly all kettlebell movements. Additionally, the squat strengthens every muscle in the lower body.

1 Standing with correct posture and with your feet shoulder width apart, flat on the floor, and pointed forward, hold the kettlebell handle with two hands comfortably in front of your body. Make sure your shoulders are pulled back and your neck is elongated. You should be looking straight ahead.

2 Lower yourself as if you were going to place the kettlebell between your legs. This should feel and look like you are sitting down on an imaginary chair. Continue until your legs form a ninety-degree angle, while your back remains straight, as if you were seated in your imaginary chair. The kettlebell should remain between your legs, and you should continue to hold it with both hands.

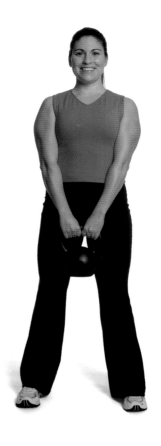

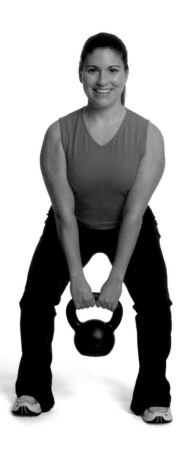

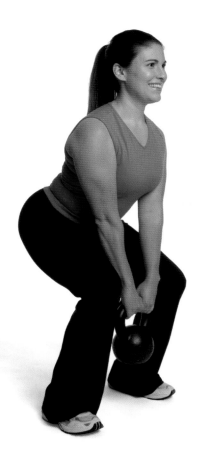

3 Return to the starting position. Be sure to check your posture to see that it's correct before attempting another repetition.

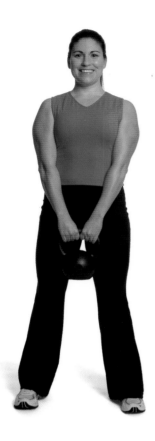

HOW MANY

2 to 3 sets for 3–5 reps for **power**, resting for 2–5 min.

2 to 3 sets for 6–8 reps for **strength**, resting for 1½–2 min.

2 to 3 sets for 8–12 reps for **growth**, resting for 1–1½ min.

2 to 3 sets for 12–20 reps for **endurance**, resting for 45 sec–1 min.

TEMPO All kettlebell movements should be performed with the intent to move quickly without compromising form or technique. **Try a tempo of 2:2**.

TO AVOID INJURY, DOUBLE-CHECK:

- Keep your feet flat on the floor.
- Be careful not to lock your knees completely.
- Maintain the natural curve of your back; avoid rounding any part of your spine.
- Make sure that your abdominal muscles are engaged throughout the movement.
- Keep your shoulders back.
- Don't flex your head forward.
- Stop lowering yourself when your legs form a ninety-degree angle, when you are positioned as if you were sitting in a chair.

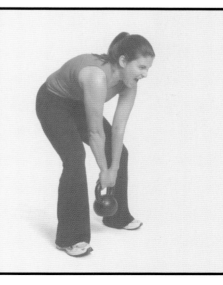

kettlebell dead lift

The dead lift is also an essential movement in a kettlebell routine. The movement will feel similar to a kettlebell squat. Instead of starting from a standing position, you will be lifting the kettlebell from the ground. Just like the squat, the dead lift also strengthens all the muscles in the lower body.

1 Start from a squat position with feet hip-width apart. The kettlebell should be on the ground between your legs, and you should be holding the handle with both hands.

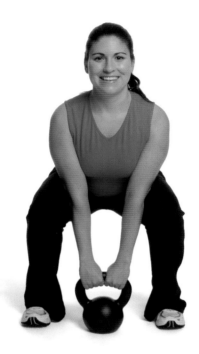

2 Begin to raise yourself to a standing position with the kettlebell handle in both hands. Keep your feet flat on the floor. Remember to maintain correct posture throughout the movement and be careful not to completely lock your knees.

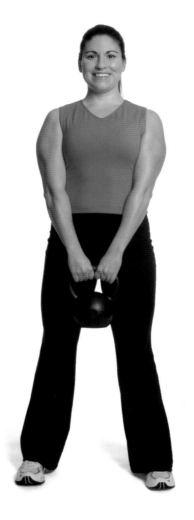

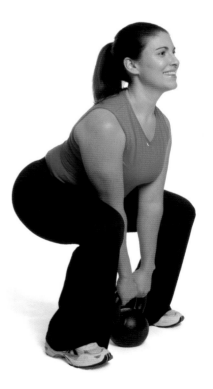

3 Return to the starting position: squatting with the kettle-bell completely on the floor between your legs. Keep both hands on the kettlebell handle, but make sure the kettlebell has made contact with the ground and has no momentum.

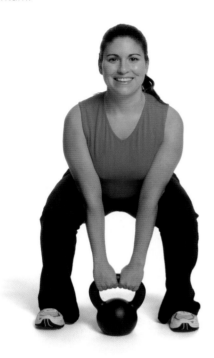

HOW MANY

2 to 3 sets for 3–5 reps for **power**, resting for 2–5 min.

2 to 3 sets for 6–8 reps for **strength**, resting for 1½–2 min.

2 to 3 sets for 8–12 reps for **growth**, resting for 1–1½ min.

2 to 3 sets for 12–20 reps for **endurance**, resting for 45 sec–1 min.

TEMPO All kettlebell movements should be performed with the intent to move quickly without compromising form or technique. **Try a tempo of 2:2.**

TO AVOID INJURY, DOUBLE-CHECK:

- Keep your feet flat on the floor.
- Be careful not to lock your knees.
- Maintain the natural curve of your back; avoid rounding at any point on your spine.
- Make sure your abdominal muscles are engaged throughout the movement.
- Keep your shoulders back.
- Don't flex your head forward.
- Keep both hands on the kettlebell throughout the movement.

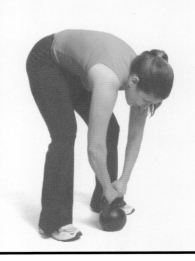

kettlebell double-arm swing squat

This exercise is a dynamic movement working both lower and upper body. The primary muscles used in the lower body are the glutes, quads, and hamstrings; the shoulders and pecs in the upper body assist with the swing.

1 Begin this movement just as if you were doing an exaggerated squat. By extending your buttocks farther back, you force your chest and torso to lean slightly forward. Firmly holding the kettlebell handle with both hands, lower your arms straight down between your legs. Remember to keep your back firm and straight.

2 Thrust your hips forward forcefully and, using the power that you generate, swing the kettlebell up, keeping your arms straight.

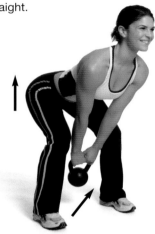

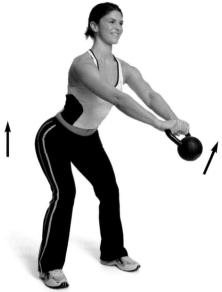

3 At this point the momentum of the swinging force will cause you to stand up straight. Your arms and kettlebell will swing up to shoulder height.

4 After reaching the zenith (the top part of the movement), gravity will cause the kettlebell and your arms to come back down the same path they came up. As this happens, you will drop back to the starting position.

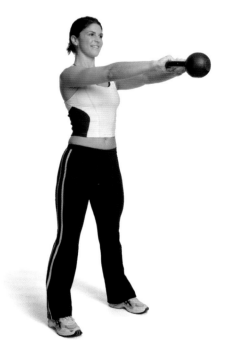

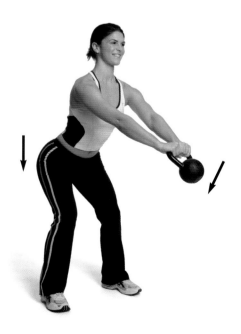

5 Gravity causes the kettlebell and your arms to come back down in the same path they came up. As this happens, you will be drop right back to the starting position. Don't resist too much, you should just be guiding the kettlebell down the path it came up. At the end of the movement you will naturally return to the starting position, ready to explode into the same motion again.

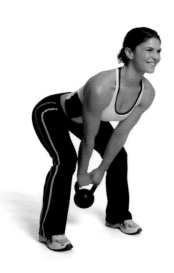

HOW MANY

2 to 3 sets for 3–5 reps for **power**, resting for 2–5 min.

2 to 3 sets for 6–8 reps for **strength**, resting for 1½–2 min.

2 to 3 sets for 8–12 reps for **growth**, resting for 1–1½ min.

2 to 3 sets for 12–20 reps for **endurance**, resting for 45 sec–1 min.

TEMPO All kettlebell movements should be performed with the intent to move quickly without compromising form or technique. **Try a tempo of 2:2 or 1:2.**

TO AVOID INJURY, DOUBLE-CHECK:

- Feet remain flat on the floor.
- Don't lock your knees completely.
- Maintain the natural curve of your back; avoid rounding any point on your spine.
- Make sure that your abdominal muscles are engaged throughout the movement.
- Keep shoulders back.
- Don't flex your head forward.
- Make sure your feet aren't spaced too far apart.
- Don't let the kettlebell dangle; you should always be in a controlled movement.

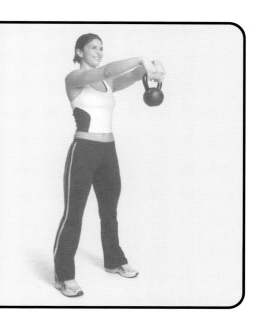

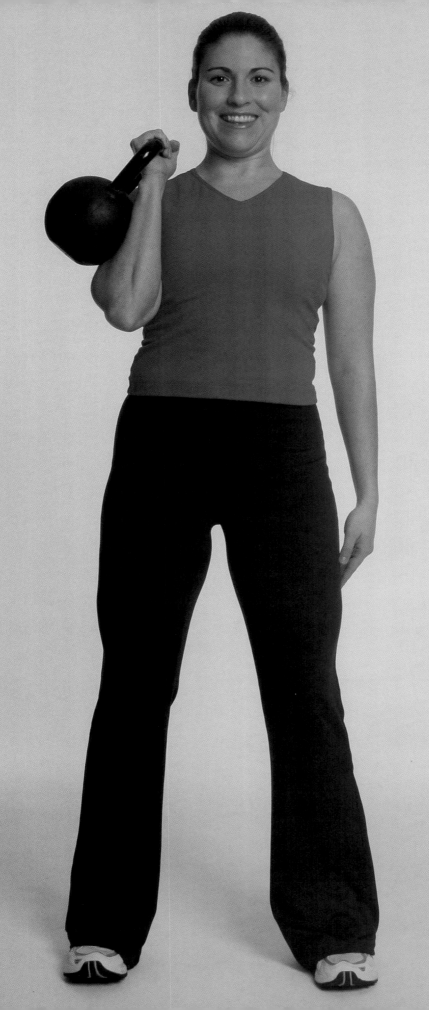

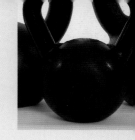

weight-lifting moves

kettlebell squat with two kettlebells

The kettlebell squat is similar to a dumbbell squat. The benefits of a squat are the strengthening and toning of the glutes, hamstrings, quads, and calf muscles. This exercise is extremely useful and should always be rotated into your workout routine.

1 Standing with correct posture with your feet shoulder width apart, flat on the floor, and pointed forward, hold each kettlebell by its handle with your arms comfortably at your sides. Pull your shoulders back and lengthen your neck. You should be looking straight ahead.

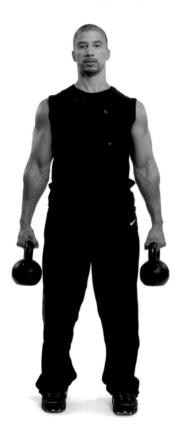
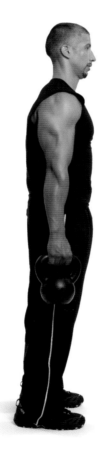

2 Lower yourself as if you were going to place the kettlebells beside your ankles. This should feel and look as if you are sitting down on a chair. Continue to lower yourself until your hips and knees are at or close to ninety-degree angles (depending on your flexibility).

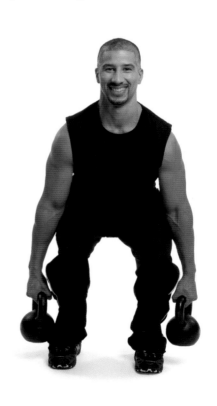
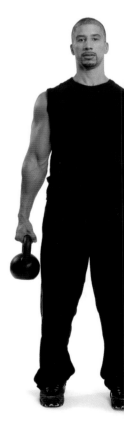

3 Return to the starting position. Be sure to check your posture before attempting another repetition.

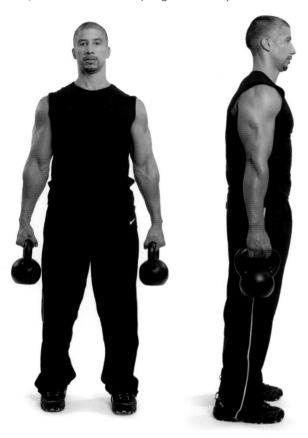

HOW MANY

2 to 3 sets for 3–5 reps for **power**, resting for 2–5 min.

2 to 3 sets for 6–8 reps for **strength**, resting for 1½–2 min.

2 to 3 sets for 8–12 reps for **growth**, resting for 1–1½ min.

2 to 3 sets for 12–20 reps for **endurance**, resting for 45 sec–1 min.

TEMPO All kettlebell movements should be performed with the intent to move quickly without compromising form or technique. **Try a tempo of 2:2**.

TO AVOID INJURY, DOUBLE-CHECK:

- Feet remain flat on the floor.
- Don't lock your knees.
- Back maintains its natural curve; avoid rounding your spine at any point.
- Make sure your abdominal muscles are engaged throughout the movement.
- Keep shoulders back.
- Don't flex your head forward.
- Remember to stop lowering yourself when you reach a ninety-degree angle between your hips and knees and you feel like you are sitting in a chair.
- Make sure your feet aren't too narrowly spaced and the kettlebells are level at your sides.

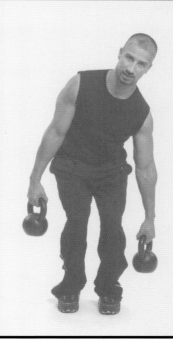

kettlebell dead lift with two kettlebells

The double kettlebell dead lift is a variation on a squat. However, because the kettlebells are starting from the floor, this move tests the flexibility of the hips. This exercise is useful and will strengthen and tone the glutes, hamstrings, quads, and calves.

1 Start from a squat position with feet hip width or farther apart. The kettlebells should be on the ground between your legs, and you should be holding a handle with each hand.

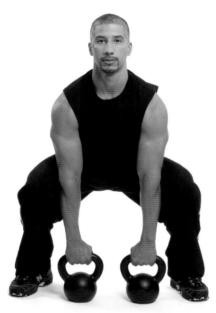

3 Stand completely erect. The kettlebells should now be in front of your thighs as you continue to hold one with each hand.

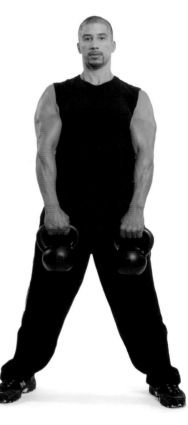

2 Begin to raise yourself to a standing position with the kettlebells between your legs. Keep your feet flat on the floor. Remember to maintain correct posture throughout the movement (chest should be facing forward).

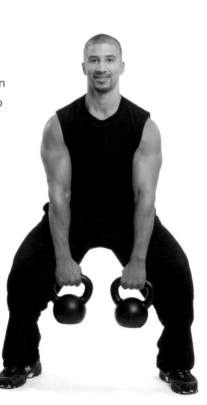

4 Return to the starting position. Make sure the kettlebell has made contact with the ground and has no momentum. Be sure to check your posture before attempting another repetition.

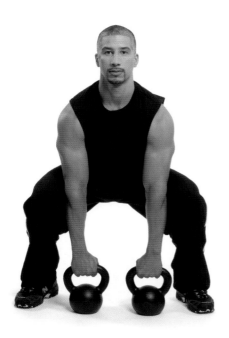

HOW MANY

2 to 3 sets for 3–5 reps for **power**, resting for 2–5 min.

2 to 3 sets for 6–8 reps for **strength**, resting for 1½–2 min.

2 to 3 sets for 8–12 reps for **growth**, resting for 1–1½ min.

2 to 3 sets for 12–20 reps for **endurance**, resting for 45 sec–1 min.

TEMPO
All kettlebell movements should be performed with the intent to move quickly without compromising form or technique. **Try a tempo of 2:2**.

TO AVOID INJURY, DOUBLE-CHECK:

- Feet remain flat on the floor.
- Don't lock your knees.
- Back maintains its natural curve; avoid rounding your spine at any point.
- Make sure your abdominal muscles are engaged throughout the movement.
- Keep shoulders back.
- Don't flex your head forward.
- Keep both hands on the kettlebell throughout the movement.

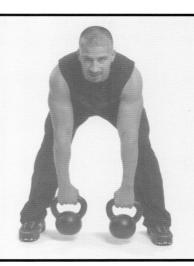

kettlebell stiff-leg dead lift

This is a single-joint movement focusing on the development of your hamstring muscles through hip extension. This movement is very important because the general population tends to have over-developed hip flexors, which creates an imbalance between the hip flexors and extensors. You should always try to keep the muscle pairs that serve a joint balanced.

1 Stand with feet flat on the floor and hip width apart. Hips are flexed to a ninety-degree angle so that your torso is parallel to the ground. Arms are parallel to your legs and both hands are holding the kettlebell. Knees should be straight.

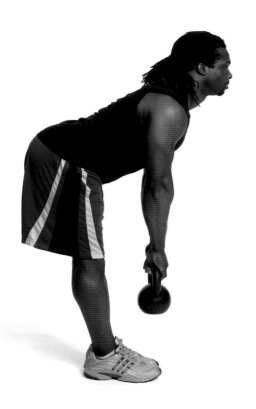

2 Move only your torso by using your hips to bring you to a standing position to complete the movement. While in the standing position, the kettlebell should be held with both hands in front of your body.

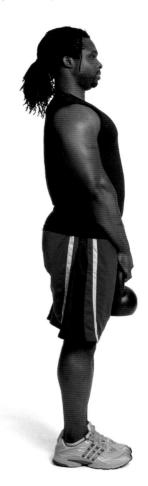

HOW MANY

2 to 3 sets for 3–5 reps for **power**, resting for 2–5 min.

2 to 3 sets for 6–8 reps for **strength**, resting for 1½–2 min.

2 to 3 sets for 8–12 reps for **growth**, resting for 1–1½ min.

2 to 3 sets for 12–20 reps for **endurance**, resting for 45 sec–1 min.

TEMPO All kettlebell movements should be performed with the intent to move quickly without compromising form or technique. **Try a tempo of 2:2**.

TO AVOID INJURY, DOUBLE-CHECK:

- Feet remain flat on the floor.
- Back maintains its natural curve; avoid rounding your spine at any point.
- Make sure your abdominal muscles are engaged throughout the movement.
- Keep shoulders back.
- Don't flex your head forward.
- Keep both hands on the kettlebell throughout the movement.

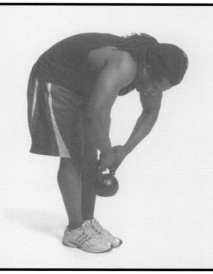

kettlebell chest press

This is a multijoint movement focusing on the development of the muscles of the chest. Secondary to the pectoral muscles, you will also be using your anterior deltoid and biceps muscles. You will need two kettlebells to perform this movement.

1 Start in a supine position (lying down on your back). Extend your arms into a T position on the ground, with your elbows flexed vertically to ninety degrees. Have a kettlebell in each hand in the rack position.

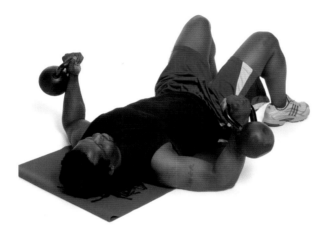

2 Press the kettlebells up, extending your elbows until your arms are straight. Palms should be facing each other and maintaining the rack grip position. As you advance, you can switch your grip to the waiter or bottoms-up position. Keep your head flat on the floor. Do not flex forward.

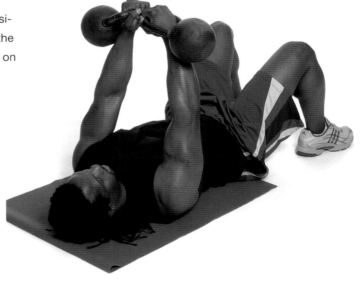

HOW MANY

2 to 3 sets for 3–5 reps for **power**, resting for 2–5 min.

2 to 3 sets for 6–8 reps for **strength**, resting for 1½–2 min.

2 to 3 sets for 8–12 reps for **growth**, resting for 1–1½ min.

2 to 3 sets for 12–20 reps for **endurance**, resting for 45 sec–1 min.

TEMPO All kettlebell movements should be performed with the intent to move quickly without compromising form or technique. **Try a tempo of 3:3.**

TO AVOID INJURY, DOUBLE-CHECK:

- Keep hips on the floor at all times.
- Engage abdominal muscles.
- Maintain proper arm position throughout the movement.
- Avoid extending your wrists too far back. Keep them in a straight line with your forearms.
- Maintain your grip on the kettlebell handle.

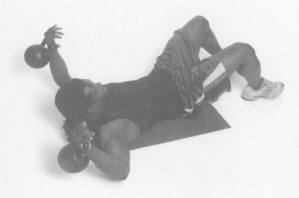
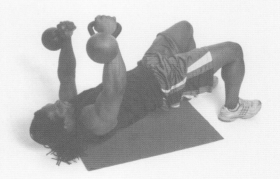

kettlebell push-ups

This is a multijoint movement focusing on strengthening the upper body. This is a great body weight exercise. This exercise can be challenging at first, but stick with it and you will see that you will be able to perform a couple more repetitions each time. It is very important to pay attention to your form in this exercise because it is very easy to develop bad habits that may be hard to break.

1 Start with your hands gripping two kettlebell handles in push-up position. Make sure your shoulders, elbows, and wrists are in one straight line and form a ninety-degree angle with the rest of your body. Your head, shoulders, hips, knees, and ankles should be in a straight line and parallel to the ground. Your feet should be hip width apart, and you should be supporting your weight on your toes and arms.

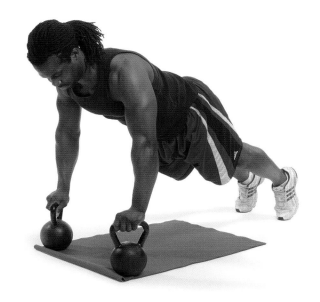

2 Lower your entire body down toward the ground, engaging all muscles in your body. Initiate the movement at your shoulders and bend your elbows, pointing them up toward the ceiling.

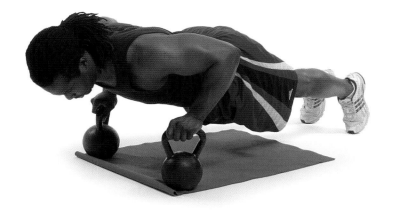

3 Push your body up and return to the starting position.

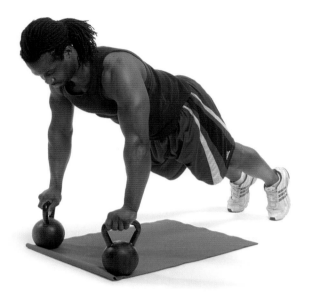

HOW MANY

2 to 3 sets for 3–5 reps for **power**, resting for 2–5 min.

2 to 3 sets for 6–8 reps for **strength**, resting for 1½–2 min.

2 to 3 sets for 8–12 reps for **growth**, resting for 1–1½ min.

2 to 3 sets for 12–20 reps for **endurance**, resting for
    45 sec–1 min.

TEMPO   This exercise does not require a quick move-ment. You are not moving the kettlebells; rather, you are stabilizing your body on top of them. You should proceed with this exercise using a slow and controlled pace, maintaining your form throughout the movement.

Try a tempo of 3:3.

TO AVOID INJURY, DOUBLE-CHECK:

- Avoid flexing or extending your head.
- Maintain a straight plank position of your body throughout the movement.
- Avoid lifting your hips when lowering your body toward the ground.
- Don't arch your back or drop your hips when lowering your body toward the ground.
- Keep your arms close to your body, allowing your elbows to point behind you, not out to the sides.
- Keep your abdominals engaged throughout the movement.

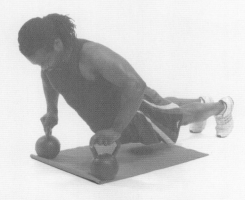
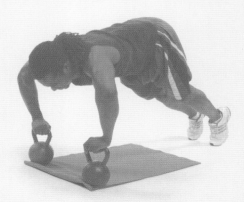

kettlebell chest fly

This is a single-joint exercise focusing on the development of the pectoral muscles. You will need two kettlebells for this exercise.

1 Start in a supine position (lying on your back). Extend your arms into a T-position on the ground with one kettle-bell in each hand.

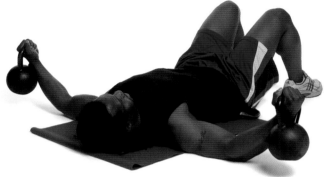

2 Maintaining the T-position with your arms, begin to bring your arms together along the horizontal plane of motion. Imagine you are hugging a beach ball.

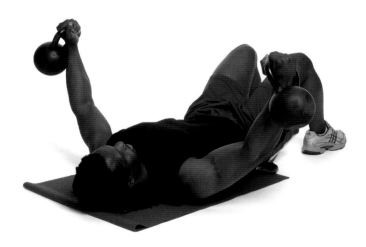

3 At the top of the arc, maintain a bowed arm position. Your palms should be facing each other with the kettle-bells in the rack position.

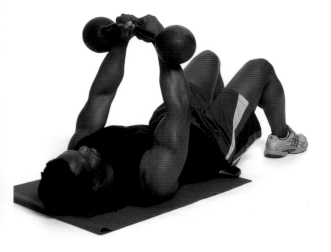

HOW MANY

2 to 3 sets for 3–5 reps for **power**, resting for 2–5 min.

2 to 3 sets for 6–8 reps for **strength**, resting for 1½–2 min.

2 to 3 sets for 8–12 reps for **growth**, resting for 1–1½ min.

2 to 3 sets for 12–20 reps for **endurance**, resting for 45 sec–1 min.

TEMPO   All kettlebell movements should be performed with the intent to move quickly without compromising form or technique. **Try a tempo of 3:3**.

TO AVOID INJURY, DOUBLE-CHECK:

- Keep head flat on the floor. Do not flex it forward.
- Keep hips on the floor at all times.
- Engage abdominal muscles.
- Maintain proper arm position throughout the movement.
- Avoid extending your wrists too far back. Keep them in a straight line with your forearms.
- Maintain your grip on the kettlebell handle.

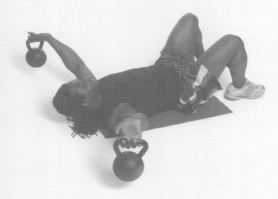

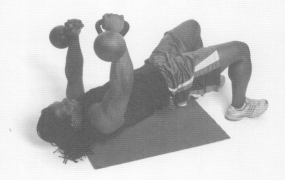

kettlebell bent-over row

This is a multijoint movement focusing on the muscles of the back and arm. Because of sitting at the computer or at a desk all day, we tend to have very rounded shoulders. This exercise will help to correct the rounded posture by strengthening the back and arm muscles.

1 Begin in a bent-knee position with your torso bent from the hips. Allow the kettlebell to be parallel to the floor.

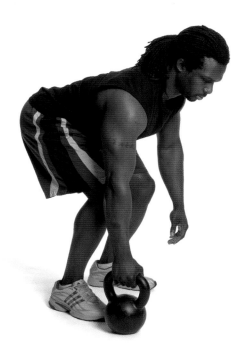

2 Initiate the movement from the shoulder by pulling the kettlebell as far as possible, allowing your elbow to bend. Feet remain flat on the floor.

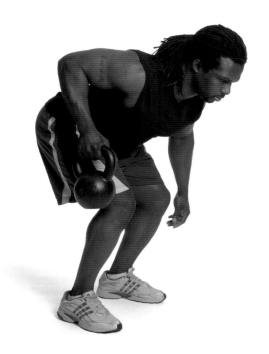

3 Return the kettlebell to the starting position.

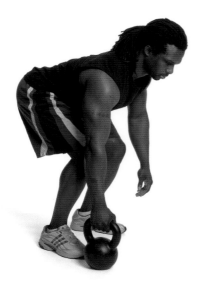

HOW MANY:

2 to 3 sets for 3–5 reps for **power**, resting for 2–5 min.

2 to 3 sets for 6–8 reps for **strength**, resting for 1½–2 min.

2 to 3 sets for 8–12 reps for **growth**, resting for 1–1½ min.

2 to 3 sets for 12–20 reps for **endurance**, resting for
   45 sec–1 min.

TEMPO All kettlebell movements should be performed with the intent to move quickly without compromising form or technique. **Try a tempo of 2:2**.

TO AVOID INJURY, DOUBLE-CHECK:

- Back maintains its natural curve; avoid rounding your spine at any point.
- Make sure your abdominal muscles are engaged throughout the movement.
- Don't flex your head forward.
- Maintain a tabletop position with your back.
- Avoid rotating your torso when pulling the kettlebell up.
- You should be looking at the ground throughout the movement.
- Maintain a straight wrist throughout the movement.

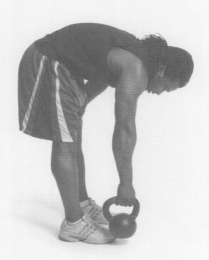

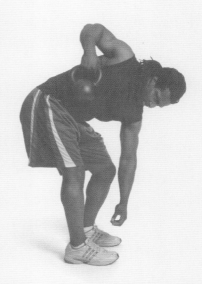

kettlebell nosebuster

This is a single-joint movement focusing on improving the strength of the triceps muscle. This tends to be an area of concern for females who are worried about the jiggle in the back of the arm. Although nutrition plays a role in body fat, increasing your lean muscle mass will certainly help burn off that unwanted back-of-the-arm jiggle. This is a great exercise to help develop the back of your arm (triceps muscle).

1 Begin in a supine position (lying flat on your back) with your upper arm off the floor and your elbow bent, holding the kettlebell handle. The kettlebell should be on the floor right by your ear.

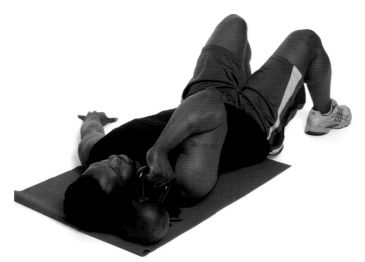

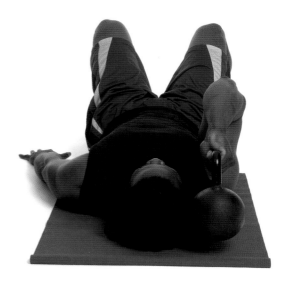

2 Extend the arm, keeping your wrist straight and bringing the kettlebell up toward the ceiling.

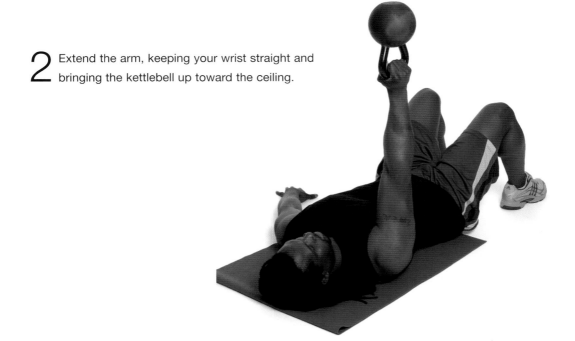

3 Return to the starting position.

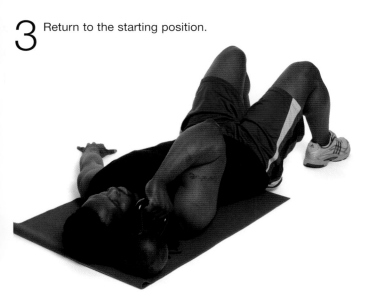

HOW MANY

2 to 3 sets for 3–5 reps for **power**, resting for 2–5 min.

2 to 3 sets for 6–8 reps for **strength**, resting for 1½–2 min.

2 to 3 sets for 8–12 reps for **growth**, resting for 1–1½ min.

2 to 3 sets for 12–20 reps for **endurance**, resting for 45 sec–1 min.

TEMPO All kettlebell movements should be performed with the intent to move quickly without compromising form or technique. **Try a tempo of 2:2.**

TO AVOID INJURY, DOUBLE-CHECK:

- Keep your head flat on the floor. Do not flex it forward.
- Keep hips on the floor at all times.
- Engage abdominal muscles.
- Maintain proper arm position throughout the movement.
- Avoid extending or flexing your wrist. Keep your wrist in a straight line with your forearm.
- Maintain your grip on the kettlebell handle.

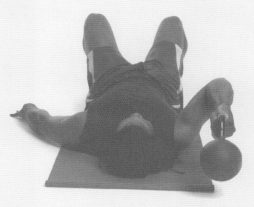

kettlebell hammer curl

This exercise works the forearm and biceps muscles. There are three muscles in your arm that help you curl/flex your arm. Using the kettlebell to do this movement makes it more demanding. The forearm and biceps muscles have to work together for the complete movement to occur.

1 Stand comfortably with feet shoulder width apart. Hold the kettle-bell firmly by its handle, letting your elbows stay at the side.

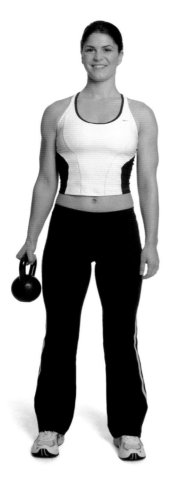

2 Curl your arm, keeping your wrist as straight as possible without moving your elbow from your side.

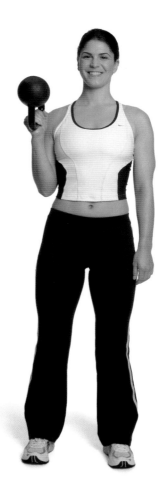

3 Slowly lower your arm back to your side (starting position).

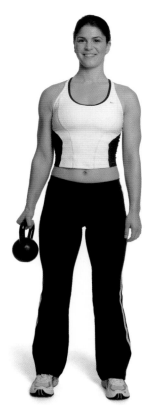

HOW MANY

2 to 3 sets for 3–5 reps for **power**, resting for 2–5 min.

2 to 3 sets for 6–8 reps for **strength**, resting for 1½–2 min.

2 to 3 sets for 8–12 reps for **growth**, resting for 1–1½ min.

2 to 3 sets for 12–20 reps for **endurance**, resting for 45 sec–1 min.

TEMPO All kettlebell movements should be performed with the intent to move quickly without compromising form or technique. **Try a tempo of 2:2 or 2:3**.

TO AVOID INJURY, DOUBLE-CHECK:

- Maintain your posture throughout the movement.
- Feet should remain flat on the floor.
- Back maintains its natural curve; avoid rounding or arching at any point during the movement.
- Make sure your abdominal muscles are engaged throughout the movement.
- Keep shoulders back.
- Don't flex your head forward.
- Maintain proper arm position throughout the movement. Avoid extending or flexing your wrist. Keep your wrist in a straight line with your forearm.
- Maintain your grip on the kettlebell handle.

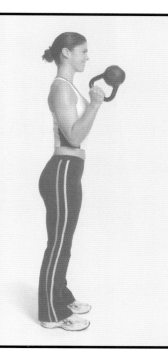

kettlebell standing unilateral (single-arm) shoulder press

This exercise uses the upper body, and if your goal is to improve your shoulder strength, this is the exercise that will do it! This exercise can be performed unilaterally (one arm) or bilaterally (two arms).

1 Stand with correct posture, feet flat on the floor and shoulder width apart. This provides a good base of support. Remember to keep your head level and look straight ahead. Choose one of the three grip positions (see pages 14–15): it is best to start with the rack position for a beginning routine. As shown here, you will start with your arm tucked close to your body. The elbow with the kettlebell should be bent and resting in the pocket between your forearm and biceps muscle.

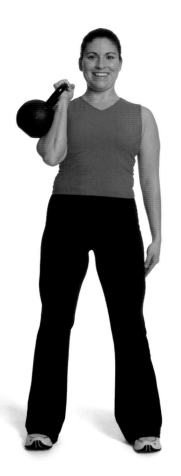

2 Raise your arm up until it is straight overhead. Keep your arm close to your ear.

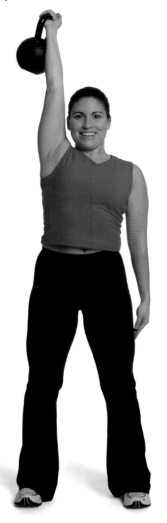

3 Return to the starting position with the kettlebell in the "pocket," in a rack position.

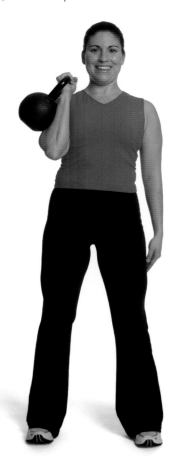

HOW MANY

2 to 3 sets for 3–5 reps for **power**, resting for 2–5 min.

2 to 3 sets for 6–8 reps for **strength**, resting for 1½–2 min.

2 to 3 sets for 8–12 reps for **growth**, resting for 1–1½ min.

2 to 3 sets for 12–20 reps for **endurance**, resting for 45 sec–1 min.

TEMPO All kettlebell movements should be performed with the intent to move quickly without compromising form or technique. **Try a tempo of 2:2.**

TO AVOID INJURY, DOUBLE-CHECK:

- Maintain your posture throughout the movement.
- Feet remain flat on the floor.
- Don't lock your knees.
- Back maintains natural curve; avoid rounding or arching at any point during the movement.
- Make sure your abdominal muscles are engaged throughout the movement.
- Keep shoulders back.
- Don't flex your head forward.

kettlebell alternating shoulder press

This exercise works the shoulder and rotator cuff muscles. Because the kettlebell's weight is on the outside of your wrist, unlike a dumbbell (with which the weight is balanced in your hand), this exercise is more challenging. Alternating the arms adds coordination and endurance training to the kettlebell shoulder press.

1 Stand with correct posture, feet flat on the floor and shoulder width apart. This allows for a good base of support. Remember to keep your head level and look straight ahead. Choose one of the three grip positions (see pages 14–15): it is best to start with the rack position for a beginning routine. As shown here, you will start with your arms tucked close to your body. The elbows with the kettlebells should be bent and resting in the pockets between your forearm and bicep muscles.

2 Raise your right arm up until it is straight overhead. Keep that arm close to or in line with your ear. The other arm should stay in the starting rack position.

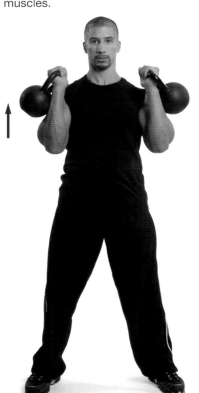

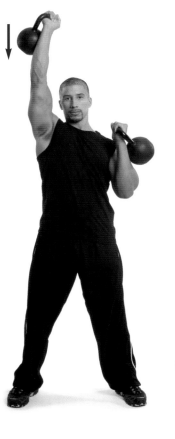

3 Bring down the right arm back to the starting rack position. Maintain your standing posture.

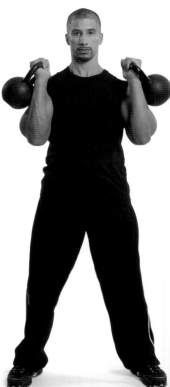

4 As soon as your right arm returns to the starting rack position, raise your left arm until it is straight overhead. Keep that arm close to or in line with your ear. The other arm should stay in the starting rack position.

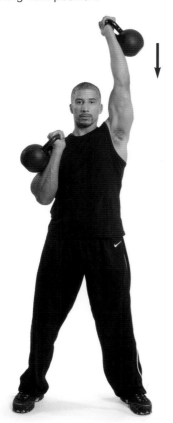

HOW MANY

2 to 3 sets for 3–5 reps for **power**, resting for 2–5 min.

2 to 3 sets for 6–8 reps for **strength**, resting for 1½–2 min.

2 to 3 sets for 8–12 reps for **growth**, resting for 1–1½ min.

2 to 3 sets for 12–20 reps for **endurance**, resting for 45 sec–1 min.

TEMPO All kettlebell movements should be performed with the intent to move quickly without compromising form or technique. **Try a tempo of 2:2.**

5 Bring the left arm back to the starting rack position. Maintain your standing posture. Continue this motion until you complete your rep range. Maintain your posture throughout the movement.

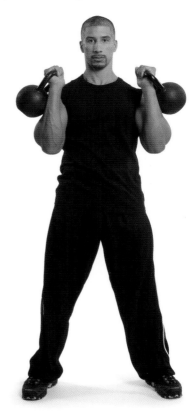

TO AVOID INJURY, DOUBLE-CHECK:

- Feet remain flat on the floor.
- Don't lock your knees.
- Back maintains its natural curve; avoid rounding or arching at any point during the movement.
- Make sure your abdominal muscles are engaged throughout the movement.
- Keep shoulders back.
- Don't flex your head forward.
- Make sure your feet aren't too close together.

kettlebell upright row

This is a multijoint movement focusing on strengthening the arms. This movement teaches you how to produce and absorb force. Most injuries occur due to the stabilizing muscles' inability to properly absorb force. This exercise can be done with one or two arms as illustrated.

KETTLEBELL UPRIGHT ROW WITH TWO ARMS

1 Begin in a standing position with your feet shoulder width apart. Hold the kettlebell handle with both hands.

2 Pull the kettlebell upward to shoulder height, keeping it close to your body. This allows the elbows to bend and point toward the ceiling.

3 Lower the kettlebell to the starting position, keeping it close to your body.

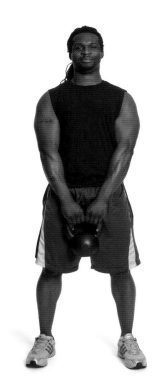
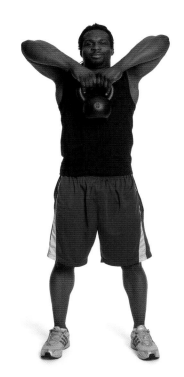

KETTLEBELL UPRIGHT ROW WITH ONE ARM

1 Begin in a standing position with your feet shoulder width apart. Hold the kettlebell handle with one hand.

2 Pull the kettlebell upward to shoulder height, keeping it close to your body. This allows the elbows to bend and point toward the ceiling.

3 Lower the kettlebell to the starting position, keeping it close to your body.

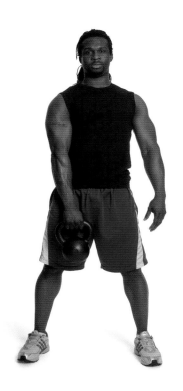
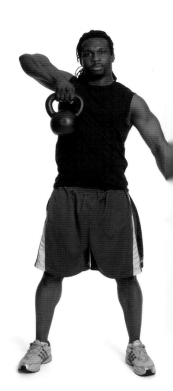

HOW MANY

2 to 3 sets for 3–5 reps for **power**, resting for 2–5 min.

2 to 3 sets for 6–8 reps for **strength**, resting for 1½–2 min.

2 to 3 sets for 8–12 reps for **growth**, resting for 1–1½ min.

2 to 3 sets for 12–20 reps for **endurance**, resting for
45 sec–1 min.

TEMPO All kettlebell movements should be performed with the intent to move quickly without compromising form or technique. **Try a tempo of 2:2.**

TO AVOID INJURY, DOUBLE-CHECK:

- Feet remain flat on the floor and shoulder width apart.
- Back maintains its natural curve; avoid rounding your spine at any point.
- Make sure your abdominal muscles are engaged throughout the movement.
- Keep shoulders back.
- Don't raise the kettlebell above shoulder height.
- Don't flex your head forward.
- Keep a good grip on the kettlebell throughout the movement.
- Look straight ahead throughout the movement.

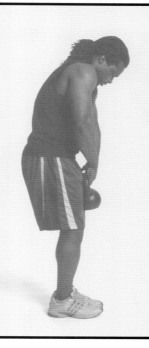

kettlebell split squat

The split squat is a lower-body stability exercise. This is a great exercise for working all the leg muscles: the quads, hamstrings, glutes, and calves. The leg that is forward does most of the work, while the back leg stabilizes your body. After mastering the basic version, you can challenge your balance by using one or two kettlebells in various grip positions. Overhead static holds will work on shoulder, elbow, and wrist stability.

1 Start this movement by spreading your feet apart: place one foot forward and the other back. The forward foot should be flat, and you should be standing on your toes with the back foot. Hold the kettlebell by your side (use one kettlebell to start, or two if you decide to challenge yourself).

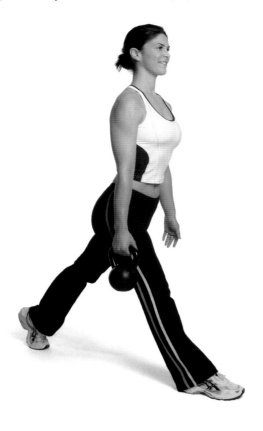

2 To start your descent, bend your back knee toward the ground. Your arms should be nice and straight as you go down and back up.

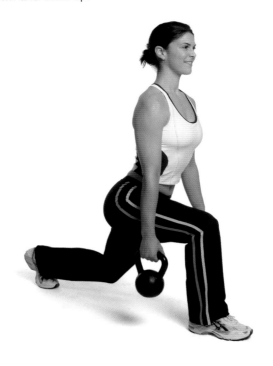

3 After you reach the bottom (end) of this movement, push downward with both legs. This will cause you to go back up to the starting position.

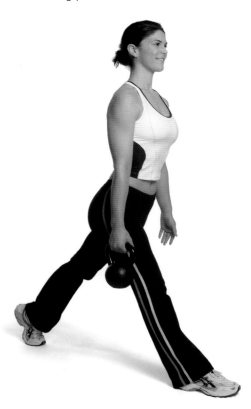

HOW MANY

2 to 3 sets for 3–5 reps for **power**, resting for 2–5 min.

2 to 3 sets for 6–8 reps for **strength**, resting for 1½–2 min.

2 to 3 sets for 8–12 reps for **growth**, resting for 1–1½ min.

2 to 3 sets for 12–20 reps for **endurance**, resting for 45 sec–1 min.

TEMPO All kettlebell movements should be performed with the intent to move quickly without compromising form or technique. **Try a tempo of 2:2 or 1:2.**

TO AVOID INJURY, DOUBLE-CHECK:

- Feet remain close enough for you to control your movement and balance.
- Make sure your feet aren't too close together.
- Make sure the heel of your front foot stays down.
- Don't lock your knees.
- Back maintains its natural curve; avoid rounding your spine at any point.
- Make sure your abdominal muscles are engaged throughout the movement.
- Keep shoulders back.
- Don't flex your head forward.

SPLIT SQUAT (BOTTOMS—UP)

1 Start this movement by spreading your feet apart: place one foot forward and the other back. The forward foot should be flat, and you should be standing on your toes with the back foot. Grip the kettlebell by its handle so the bottom of the kettlebell is facing the ceiling. (Use one kettlebell on either side, or hold two kettlebells at the same time if you decide to challenge yourself.) Hold the kettlebell overhead with a straight arm.

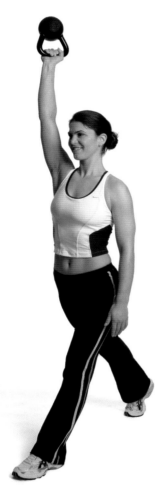

2 To start your descent, bend your back knee toward the ground. The challenge will be to keep the kettlebell and arm straight while in the bottoms-up position.

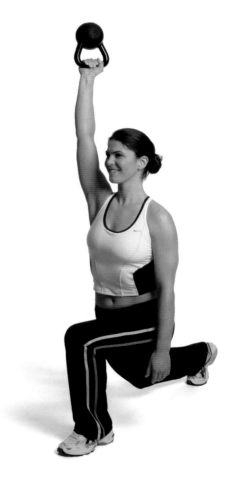

3 After you reach the bottom (end) of the movement, push downward with both legs, causing you to rise back up to the starting position.

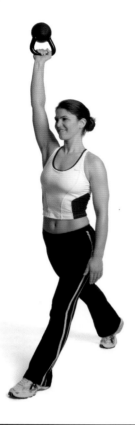

HOW MANY

2 to 3 sets for 3–5 reps for **power**, resting for 2–5 min.

2 to 3 sets for 6–8 reps for **strength**, resting for 1½–2 min.

2 to 3 sets for 8–12 reps for **growth**, resting for 1–1½ min.

2 to 3 sets for 12–20 reps for **endurance**, resting for 45 sec–1 min.

TEMPO All kettlebell movements should be performed with the intent to move quickly without compromising form or technique. **Try a tempo of 2:2 or 1:2.**

TO AVOID INJURY, DOUBLE-CHECK:

- Feet remain close enough together to control movement and balance.
- Make sure your feet aren't too close together.
- Make sure your front foot's heel stays down.
- Don't lock your knees.
- Back maintains its natural curve; avoid rounding your spine at any point.
- Make sure your abdominal muscles are engaged throughout the movement.
- Keep shoulders back.
- Don't flex your head forward.
- Kettlebell arm should be straight and close to or in line with your ear.
- Don't lean too far over the front leg.

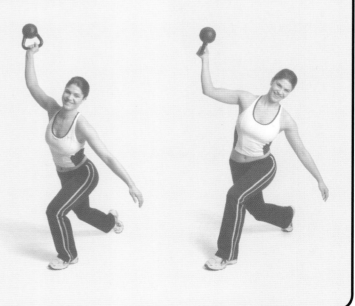

kettlebell step-back lunge (rack position)

The step back lunge is another variation of lunging. Stepping backward improves your balance and weight distribution and targets all the muscles of the legs. This lunge challenges the stability of your front leg while stepping backward.

1 Start this movement by standing up straight with both feet together. Hold the kettlebell in the rack position. The elbow with the kettlebell should be held firmly against the side of your body.

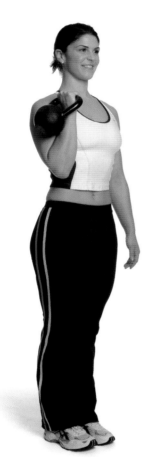

2 As you step back to a comfortable distance behind you, simultaneously begin to push the kettlebell upward. The grounded leg will be forced to support and balance your body.

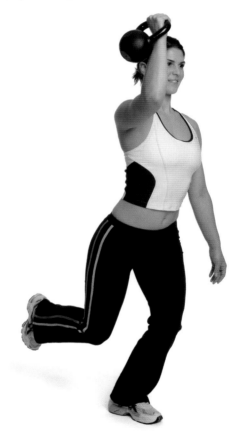

3 You'll land in the bottom or end phase of a split squat, with the kettlebell over your head.

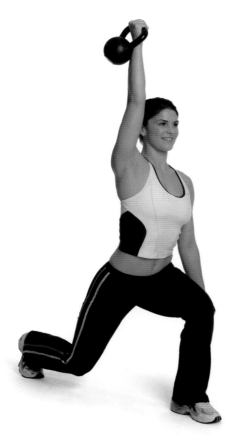

4 To return to the starting position, simultaneously push your lower body up and forward, and bring the kettlebell into the starting rack position.

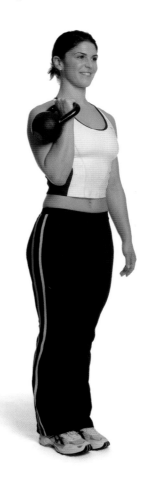

kettlebell step-forward lunge

The forward lunge is a lower-body transport exercise that works on producing and absorbing force. The lower body is challenged by having to accelerate and decelerate the force it produces. The leg that lunges forward does the majority of the work. A forward lunge is a great exercise to work the lower body.

1 Start this movement by standing up straight with both feet together. Hold the kettlebell in the rack position; remember that the elbow with the kettlebell stays firmly on the side of your body.

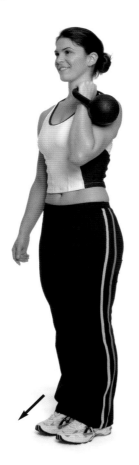

2 Pick a spot and, using your left or right foot, step forward to a comfortable distance. As you do this, you'll land in the bottom or end phase of a split squat.

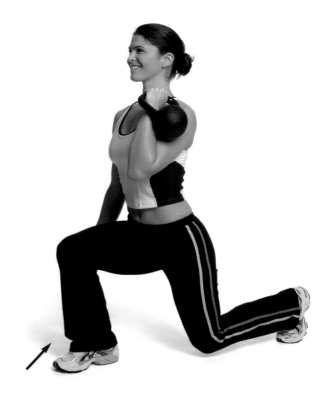

3 Just apply a reverse backward force to push yourself upward to the starting position. The arm with the kettle-bell does not move.

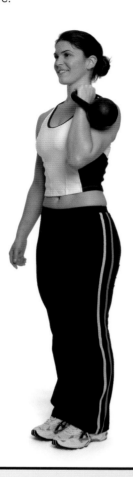

HOW MANY

2 to 3 sets for 3–5 reps for **power**, resting for 2–5 min.

2 to 3 sets for 6–8 reps for **strength**, resting for 1½–2 min.

2 to 3 sets for 8–12 reps for **growth**, resting for 1–1½ min.

2 to 3 sets for 12–20 reps for **endurance**, resting for 45 sec–1 min.

TEMPO All kettlebell movements should be performed with the intent to move quickly without compromising form or technique. **Try a tempo of 2:2 or 1:2.**

TO AVOID INJURY, DOUBLE-CHECK:

- Use the lunging foot to shoot for a manageable distance.
- Make sure your feet aren't too close together.
- Make sure your front heel stays down.
- Don't lock your knees.
- Back maintains its natural curve; avoid rounding your spine at any point.
- Make sure your abdominal muscles are engaged throughout the movement.
- Keep shoulders back.
- Don't flex your head forward.
- Make sure the arm with the kettlebell does not move.

kettlebell step-forward pickups

A step-forward pickup lunge is mainly a lower-body exercise. The glutes, quads, hamstrings, and calves will be working to perform it. Because you pick up the kettlebell from the ground, your core will stabilize in order to maintain balance. This exercise is a deep lunge, making it more challenging.

1 Start by standing up straight with your feet together. Place the kettle-bell on the ground at a comfortable lunging distance away from you. The kettlebell should be placed to the side of the hand that will be picking it up.

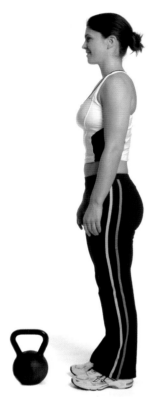

2 Lunge forward with the right foot, reaching for the kettlebell with your left arm. Get a firm grip on the handle.

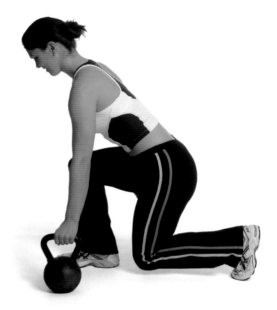

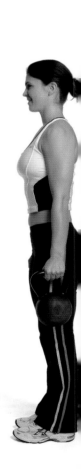

3 Push yourself back up into a standing position with the kettlebell by your side.

4 Return the kettlebell to the ground the same way you picked it up, by lunging forward with the right foot and placing down the kettlebell with your left arm.

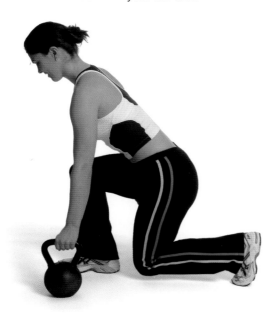

5 Push yourself up to the standing position, leaving the kettlebell on the ground.

HOW MANY

2 to 3 sets for 3–5 reps for **power**, resting for 2–5 min.

2 to 3 sets for 6–8 reps for **strength**, resting for 1$\frac{1}{2}$–2 min.

2 to 3 sets for 8–12 reps for **growth**, resting for 1–1$\frac{1}{2}$ min.

2 to 3 sets for 12–20 reps for **endurance**, resting for 45 sec–1 min.

TEMPO All kettlebell movements should be performed with the intent to move quickly without compromising form or technique. **Try a tempo of 2:2 or 1:2.**

TO AVOID INJURY, DOUBLE-CHECK:

- Bend your knees, not your back.
- Back maintains its natural curve; avoid rounding your spine at any point.
- Make sure your abdominal muscles are engaged throughout the movement.
- Keep shoulders back.
- Don't flex your head forward.
- Make sure your feet aren't too close together.

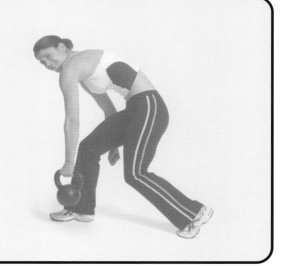

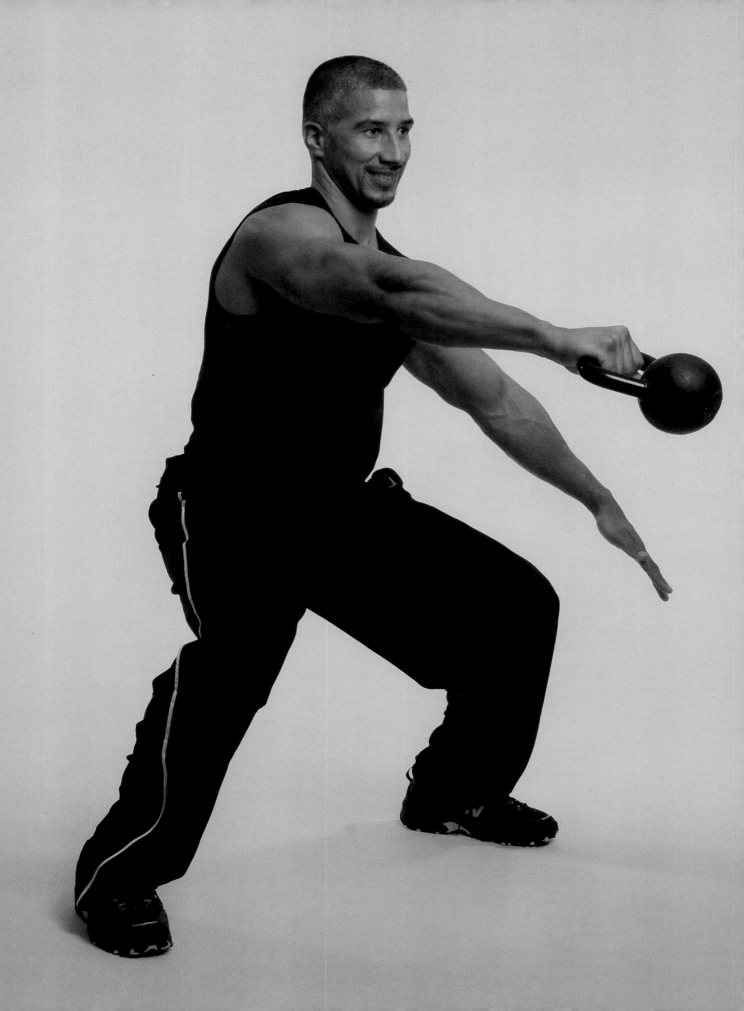

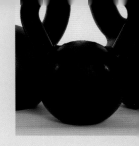

momentum moves

kettlebell double- and single-arm high pull

This multijoint movement strengthens the entire body. This exercise is a progression of the upright row (see pages 46–47). The differences between the upright row and the high pull are the use of momentum, the absorption of the momentum, and the starting position—the kettlebell is on the ground. This exercise can be performed bilaterally (double arm) or unilaterally (single arm).

KETTLEBELL DOUBLE-ARM HIGH PULL

1 Begin in a lowered squat position with both hands comfortably holding the kettlebell handle.

2 Push off the ground, distributing your weight evenly along your feet, to a standing position. Allow the kettlebell to rise quickly to shoulder height, as in an upright row. Ideally, you want to produce enough momentum with your squat to facilitate the upright row.

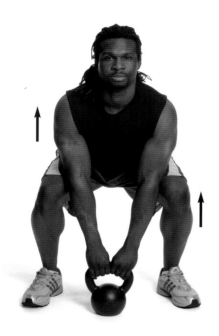

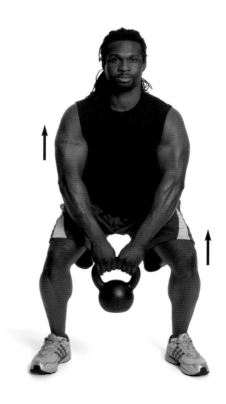

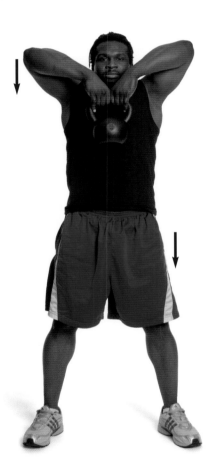

3 Absorb the momentum by allowing gravity and the weight of the kettlebell to place you back in the starting position.

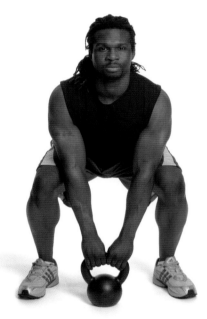

KETTLEBELL SINGLE-ARM HIGH PULL

1 Begin in a lowered squat position, holding the kettlebell handle comfortably with one hand.

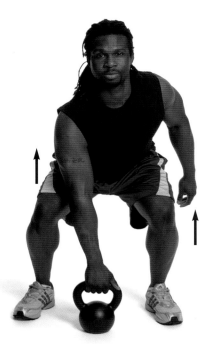

2 Push off the ground, distributing your weight evenly along your feet, to a standing position. Allow the kettlebell to rise quickly to shoulder height, as in an upright row. Ideally, you want to produce enough momentum with your squat to facilitate the upright row.

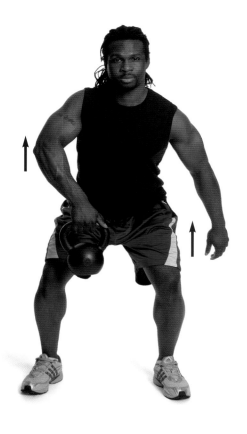

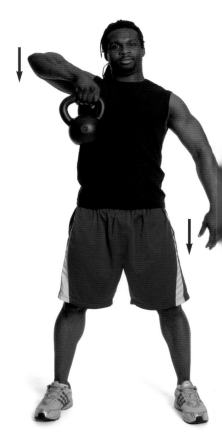

3 Absorb the momentum by allowing gravity and the weight of the kettlebell to place you back in the starting position.

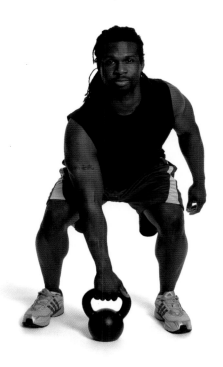

HOW MANY

2 to 3 sets for 3–5 reps for **power**, resting for 2–5 min.

2 to 3 sets for 6–8 reps for **strength**, resting for 1½–2 min.

2 to 3 sets for 8–12 reps for **growth**, resting for 1–1½ min.

2 to 3 sets for 12–20 reps for **endurance**, resting for 45 sec–1 min.

TEMPO All kettlebell movements should be performed with the intent to move quickly without compromising form or technique. **Try a tempo of 2:2**.

TO AVOID INJURY, DOUBLE-CHECK:

- Feet remain flat on the floor and shoulder width apart.
- Back maintains its natural curve; avoid rounding your spine at any point.
- Make sure your abdominal muscles are engaged throughout the movement.
- Keep shoulders back.
- Avoid raising the kettlebell above shoulder height.
- Don't flex your head forward.
- Keep a good grip on the kettlebell throughout the movement
- Look straight ahead throughout the movement.

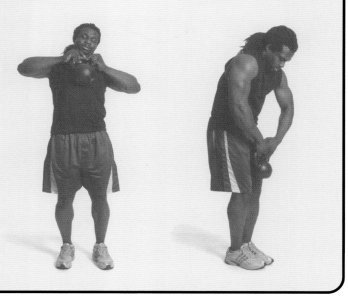

kettlebell push press

This is a more dynamic shoulder press that requires using the speed of the lower and upper body. By incorporating the use of a squat, you generate enough force to lift heavier weights overhead. This exercise works the entire body.

1 Choose one of the three grip positions (see pages 14–15). It is best to start with the rack position for a beginning routine, which we will illustrate here. Start with the kettlebell in the rack position with the kettlebell between your forearm and biceps. Sit into a quarter squat position with your feet spaced at a comfortable distance apart. Keep your head straight, and place your free arm anywhere for balance.

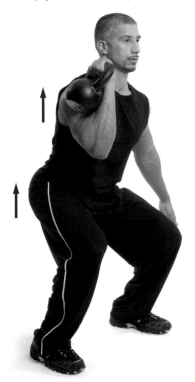

2 Begin to force yourself up into a standing position, while simultaneously driving the kettlebell up off your biceps but still keeping it in contact with your forearm. Your feet should be flat on the ground and your head should be facing forward.

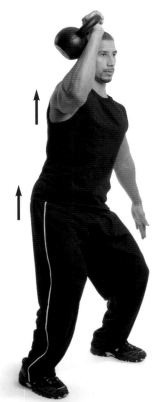

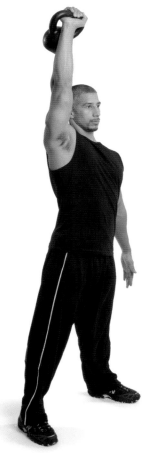

3 The force will carry you into a standing position with the kettlebell held over your head with a straight arm. The kettlebell arm should be close to or in line with your ears.

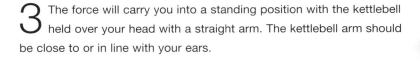

4 Return to the starting position the same way you came up. Start to drop your kettlebell arm and hips until you are back in the starting position.

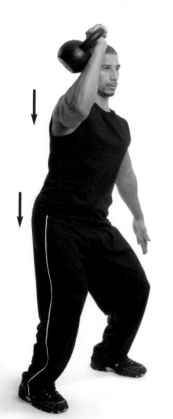
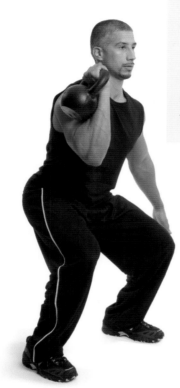

HOW MANY

2 to 3 sets for 3–5 reps for **power**, resting for 2–5 min.

2 to 3 sets for 6–8 reps for **strength**, resting for 1½–2 min.

2 to 3 sets for 8–12 reps for **growth**, resting for 1–1½ min.

2 to 3 sets for 12–20 reps for **endurance**, resting for 45 sec–1 min.

TEMPO All kettlebell movements should be performed with the intent to move quickly without compromising form or technique. **Try a tempo of 2:2 or 1:2.**

TO AVOID INJURY, DOUBLE-CHECK:

- Feet remain flat on the floor.
- Don't lock your knees.
- Back maintains its natural curve; avoid rounding your spine at any point.
- Make sure your abdominal muscles are engaged throughout the movement.
- Keep shoulders back.
- Don't flex your head forward.
- Make sure your feet aren't too close together.

kettlebell push jerk

This exercise is very complex. As in the push press (see pages 64–65), there is an added squat, which assists you in lifting even heavier weights overhead. This movement happens very quickly, so the challenge is to coordinate each phase in sequence. The use of your lower body and the speed at which you release upward from your squat allow this lift to occur.

1 Choose one of the three grip positions (see pages 14–15). It is best to use the rack position for a beginning routine, which we will illustrate here. Start with the kettlebell in the rack position with the kettlebell tucked between your forearm and biceps. Sit into a quarter squat position with your feet spaced at a comfortable distance apart. Keep your head straight and place your free arm anywhere for balance.

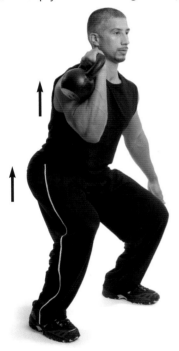

2 Begin to force yourself up into a standing position, simultaneously driving the kettlebell up off your biceps but keeping it in contact with your forearm. Your feet should still be flat on the ground and your head should be facing forward.

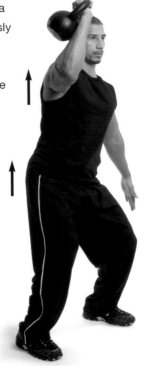

3 The force will carry you into an almost-standing position with the kettlebell over your head and with a straight arm. The trick here is to drop into a squat quickly as you straighten your arm up over your head.

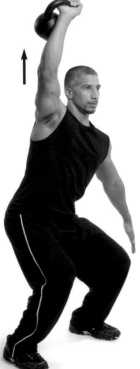

4 Keep your arm straight over your head, then stand up.

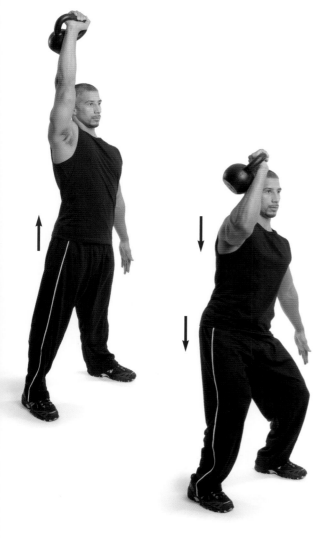

HOW MANY

2 to 3 sets for 3–5 reps for **power**, resting for 2–5 min.

2 to 3 sets for 6–8 reps for **strength**, resting for 1½–2 min.

2 to 3 sets for 8–12 reps for **growth**, resting for 1–1½ min.

2 to 3 sets for 12–20 reps for **endurance**, resting for 45 sec–1 min.

TEMPO All kettlebell movements should be performed with the intent to move quickly without compromising form or technique. **Try a tempo of 2:2 or 1:2.**

5 Return to the starting position. Start to drop your kettlebell arm, buttocks, and hips until you are back in the starting position.

TO AVOID INJURY, DOUBLE-CHECK:

- Feet remain flat on the floor.
- Don't lock your knees.
- Back maintains its natural curve; avoid rounding your spine at any point.
- Make sure your abdominal muscles are engaged throughout the movement.
- Keep shoulders back.
- Don't flex your head forward.
- Make sure the space between your feet isn't too narrow.

kettlebell single-arm swing squat

This exercise is a dynamic movement working both the lower and upper body. The primary movers of the lower body are the glutes, quads, and hamstrings, while the shoulders and pecs in the upper body assist with the swing.

1 Begin this movement just as if you were doing an exaggerated squat. By extending your buttocks farther back, you force a slight forward lean in your chest and torso. Firmly holding the kettlebell handle with one hand, lower your arm straight down between your legs. Remember to keep your back firm and straight.

2 Thrust your hips forward forcefully and, using the power that you generate, swing the kettlebell up, keeping your arm straight.

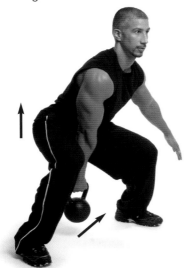

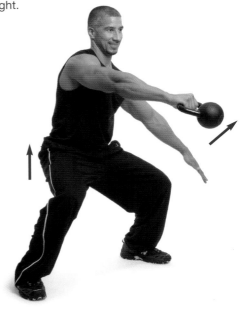

3 At this point, the momentum of the swinging force will cause you to stand up straight. Your arm and kettlebell will swing up to shoulder height.

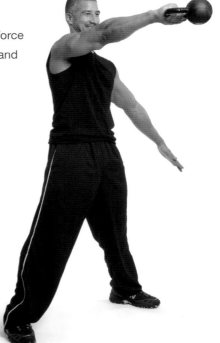

4 After reaching the zenith (the top part of the movement), gravity will cause the kettlebell and your arm to come back down the same path they came up. As this happens, you will be dropping right back to the starting position. Don't resist too much; you should just be guiding the kettlebell down the path it came up.

HOW MANY

2 to 3 sets for 3–5 reps for **power**, resting for 2–5 min.

2 to 3 sets for 6–8 reps for **strength**, resting for 1½–2 min.

2 to 3 sets for 8–12 reps for **growth**, resting for 1–1½ min.

2 to 3 sets for 12–20 reps for **endurance**, resting for 45 sec–1 min.

TEMPO All kettlebell movements should be performed with the intent to move quickly without compromising form or technique. **Try a tempo of 2:2 or 1:2.**

5 At the end of the movement, you will fall right back into the starting position, ready to start the same explosive motions again.

TO AVOID INJURY, DOUBLE-CHECK:

- Feet remain flat on the floor.
- Don't lock your knees.
- Back maintains its natural curve; avoid rounding your spine at any point.
- Make sure your abdominal muscles are engaged throughout the movement.
- Keep shoulders back.
- Don't flex your head forward.
- Make sure your feet aren't too close together.
- Don't let the kettlebell dangle at any time.

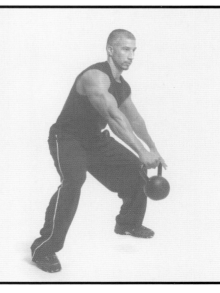

kettlebell alternating swing squat

This exercise is a variation of the single-arm swing squat (see pages 68–69). It works on timing and motor skills, making it a difficult yet fun challenge. Because you will be changing the kettlebell from hand to hand quickly, your heart rate will elevate rapidly, making this a great challenge to your cardiovascular system. This exercise will strengthen and increase endurance in all your muscles.

1 Begin this movement just as if you were doing an exaggerated squat. By extending your buttocks farther back, you force a slight forward lean in your chest and torso. Firmly holding the kettlebell handle with one hand, lower your arm straight down between your legs. Remember to keep your back firm and straight.

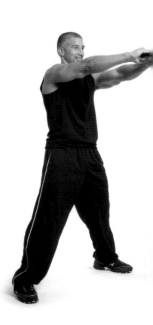

2 Thrust your hips forward forcefully and, using the power that you generate, swing the kettlebell up, keeping your arm straight.

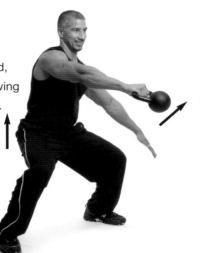

3 At this point, the momentum of the swinging force will cause you to stand up straight. Your arm and kettlebell will swing up to shoulder height.

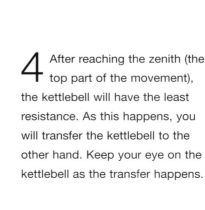

4 After reaching the zenith (the top part of the movement), the kettlebell will have the least resistance. As this happens, you will transfer the kettlebell to the other hand. Keep your eye on the kettlebell as the transfer happens.

5 Gravity will cause the kettlebell and your arms to come back down the same path they came up. As this happens, you will be dropping back to the starting position. Don't resist too much; you should just be guiding the kettlebell down the path by which it came up.

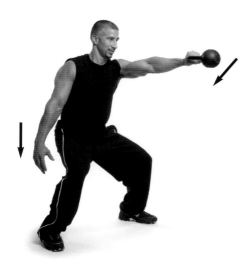

HOW MANY

2 to 3 sets for 3–5 reps for **power**, resting for 2–5 min.

2 to 3 sets for 6–8 reps for **strength**, resting for 1½–2 min.

2 to 3 sets for 8–12 reps for **growth**, resting for 1–1½ min.

2 to 3 sets for 12–20 reps for **endurance**, resting for 45 sec–1 min.

TEMPO All kettlebell movements should be performed with the intent to move quickly without compromising form or technique. **Try a tempo of 2:2 or 1:2**.

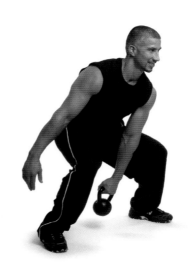

6 At the end of the movement return to the starting position, but with the kettlebell in the other hand, ready to start the same explosive motions again.

TO AVOID INJURY, DOUBLE-CHECK:

- Feet remain flat on the floor.
- Don't lock your knees.
- Back maintains its natural curve; avoid rounding your spine at any point.
- Make sure your abdominal muscles are engaged throughout the movement.
- Keep shoulders back.
- Don't flex your head forward.
- Make sure your feet aren't too close together.

kettlebell swing clean

A kettlebell swing clean is a power exercise. Power movements are fun because they move quickly and focus on multitasking. All the muscles of the body are activated when performing this movement. Another component to a swing clean is the finishing movement, which works on decelerating the kettlebell by using your hand grip to slow it down.

1 Begin this movement just as if you were doing an exaggerated squat. By extending your buttocks farther back, you force a slight forward lean in your chest and torso. Firmly holding the kettlebell handle with one hand, lower your arm straight down between your legs. Remember to keep your back firm and straight.

2 Thrust your hips forward forcefully and, using the power that you generate, swing the kettlebell up, keeping your arm straight.

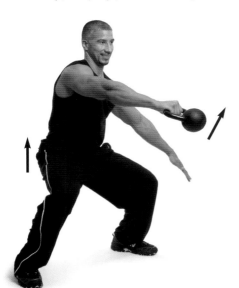

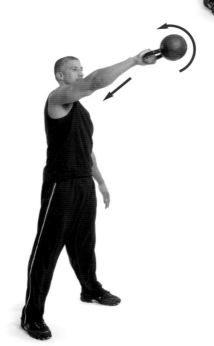

3 At this point, the momentum of the swinging force will cause you to stand up straight. Your arm and the kettlebell will swing up slightly higher than shoulder height. Give the kettlebell a slight tug toward your body.

4 The tug will cause the kettlebell to take a different path. Direct it to come down between your forearm and biceps (the rack position); at the same time, begin to lower your body to absorb the impact of the kettlebell.

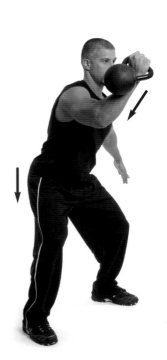

5 The resulting movement will look like the kettlebell push jerk (see page 66) starting position. The kettlebell is in the rack position between your forearm and biceps, and you are sitting in a quarter squat position with your feet spaced comfortably apart, your head straight, and your free arm placed anywhere for balance.

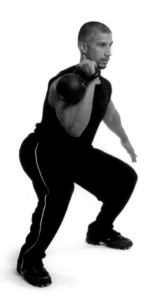

HOW MANY

2 to 3 sets for 3–5 reps for **power**, resting for 2–5 min.

2 to 3 sets for 6–8 reps for **strength**, resting for 1½–2 min.

2 to 3 sets for 8–12 reps for **growth**, resting for 1–1½ min.

2 to 3 sets for 12–20 reps for **endurance**, resting for 45 sec–1 min.

TEMPO All kettlebell movements should be performed with the intent to move quickly without compromising form or technique. **Try a tempo of 2:2 or 1:2.**

6 To return to the starting position, thrust your hips upward to the standing position while pushing the kettlebell away from your body. Let the momentum take the kettlebell down between your legs.

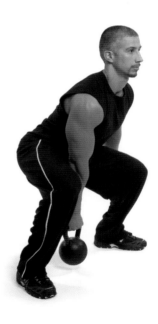

TO AVOID INJURY, DOUBLE-CHECK:

- Feet remain flat on the floor.
- Don't lock your knees.
- Back maintains its natural curve; avoid rounding your spine at any point.
- Make sure your abdominal muscles are engaged throughout the movement.
- Keep shoulders back.
- Don't flex your head forward.
- Make sure your feet aren't too close together.

kettlebell swing clean with push press

A swing clean into a push press increases the workload on the shoulder and pectoral muscles. These movements are both power exercises. Performed together, they will increase your body's ability to multitask, move quickly, and endure. Your entire body and musculature will work to maintain the sequence of this combination.

1 Begin this movement just as if you were doing an exaggerated squat. By extending your buttocks farther back, you force a slight forward lean in your chest and torso. Firmly holding the kettle-bell handle with one hand, lower your arm straight down between your legs. Remember to keep your back firm and straight.

2 Thrust your hips forward forcefully and, using the power that you generate, swing the kettlebell up, keeping your arm straight.

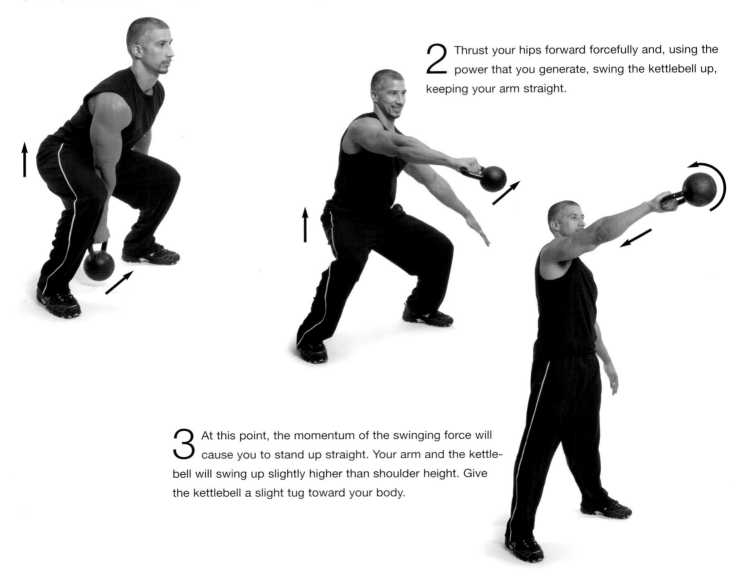

3 At this point, the momentum of the swinging force will cause you to stand up straight. Your arm and the kettle-bell will swing up slightly higher than shoulder height. Give the kettlebell a slight tug toward your body.

4 The tug will cause the kettlebell to take a different path.
Direct it to come down between your forearm and biceps
(the rack position); at the same time, begin to lower your body
to absorb the impact of the kettlebell.

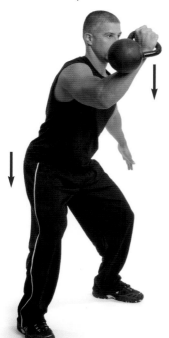

5 The resulting movement will look like the push
jerk (page 66) starting position. The kettlebell is in
the rack position between your forearm and biceps,
and you are sitting in a quarter squat position with your
feet spaced comfortably apart, your head straight, and
your free arm placed anywhere for balance.

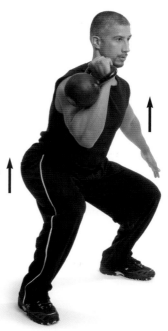

6 Begin to force yourself up into a standing
position, simultaneously driving the
kettlebell up off your biceps but keeping it in
contact with your forearm. Your feet should be
flat on the ground and your head should be
facing forward.

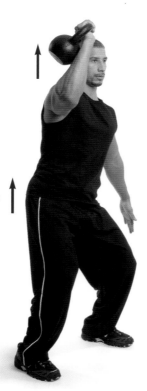

7 The force will carry you into a standing position holding the kettlebell
over your head with a straight arm. The kettlebell arm should be close
to or in line with your ears.

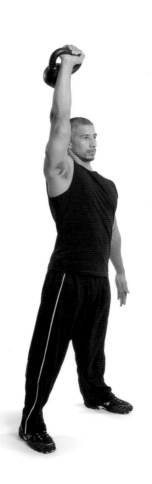

8 Return to the starting position the same way you came up. Start to drop your kettlebell arm, buttocks, and hips until you are back in the push press starting position.

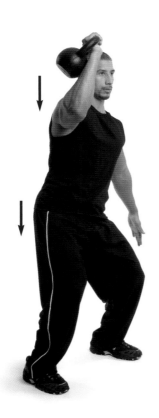

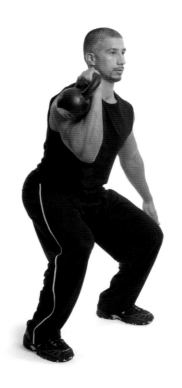

9 To return to the starting position, thrust your hips upward to the standing position while pushing the kettlebell away from your body. Let the momentum take the kettlebell down between your legs.

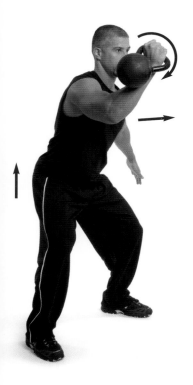

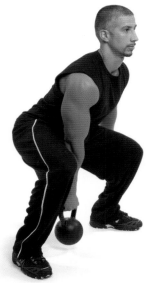

HOW MANY

2 to 3 sets for 3–5 reps for **power**, resting for 2–5 min.

2 to 3 sets for 6–8 reps for **strength**, resting for 1½–2 min.

2 to 3 sets for 8–12 reps for **growth**, resting for 1–1½ min.

2 to 3 sets for 12–20 reps for **endurance**, resting for 45 sec–1 min.

TEMPO All kettlebell movements should be performed with the intent to move quickly without compromising form or technique. **Try a tempo of 2:2 or 1:2.**

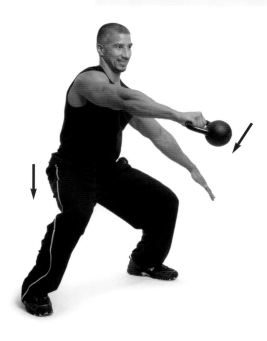

TO AVOID INJURY, DOUBLE-CHECK:

- Feet remain flat on the floor.
- Don't lock your knees.
- Back maintains its natural curve; avoid rounding your spine at any point.
- Make sure your abdominal muscles are engaged throughout the movement.
- Keep shoulders back.
- Don't flex your head forward.
- Make sure your feet aren't too close together.

kettlebell swing clean with push jerk

This combination is similar to the swing clean with push press (see pages 74–77); however, it is slightly more challenging and can be performed with a heavier kettlebell. More power and speed will be required because of the heavier kettlebell and the push jerk. This exercise will allow you to concentrate on practicing explosive movements. Remember to always allow enough rest between sets. Because these exercises are complex, they will be both physically and mentally challenging.

1 Begin this movement just as if you were doing an exaggerated squat. By extending your buttocks farther back,
you force a slight forward lean in your chest and torso. Firmly
holding the kettlebell handle with one hand, lower that arm
straight down between your legs. Remember to keep your
back firm and straight.

2 Thrust your hips forward forcefully and, using the
power that you generate, swing the kettlebell up,
keeping your arm straight.

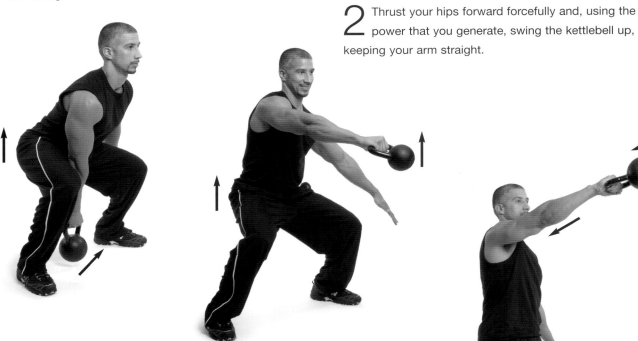

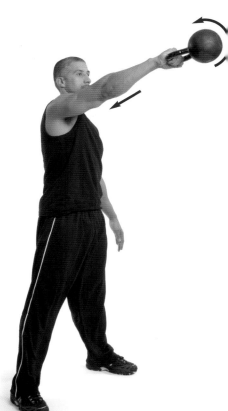

3 At this point, the momentum of the swinging force will
cause you to stand up straight. Your arm and the kettlebell
will swing up slightly higher than shoulder height. Give the
kettlebell a slight tug toward your body.

4 The tug will cause the kettlebell to take a different path. Direct it to come down between your forearm and biceps (the rack position); at the same time, begin to lower your body to absorb the impact of the kettlebell.

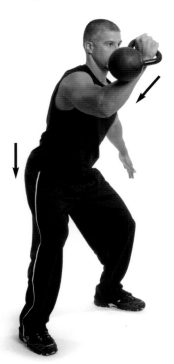

5 The resulting movement will look like the push jerk (page 66) starting position. The kettlebell is in the rack position between your forearm and biceps, and you are sitting in a quarter squat position with your feet spaced comfortably apart, your head straight, and your free arm placed anywhere for balance.

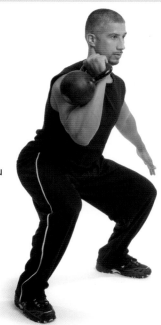

6 Begin to force yourself up into a standing position, simultaneously driving the kettlebell up off your biceps but remaining in contact with your forearm. Your feet should still be flat on the ground, and your head should be facing forward.

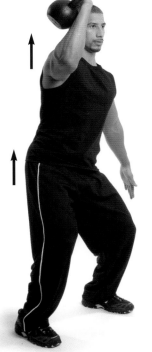

7 The force will carry you into an almost-standing position with the kettlebell held over your head with a straight arm. The trick here is to drop into a squat quickly as you straighten your arm up over your head.

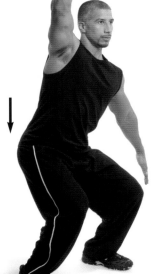

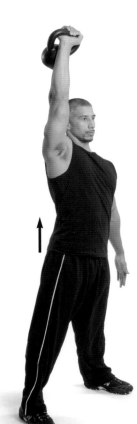

8 Keep your arm held straight over your head as you stand up.

9 Return to the starting position the same way you came up. Start
to drop your kettlebell arm, buttocks, and hips until you are back
in the push press starting position.

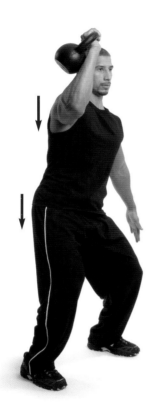

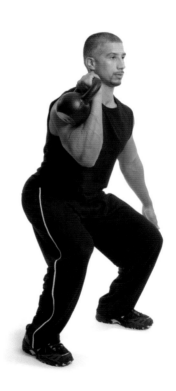

10 To return to the start position of this movement, thrust your hips upward to the standing position while pushing the kettlebell away from your body. Let the momentum take the kettlebell back down between your legs.

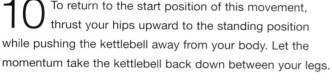

HOW MANY

2 to 3 sets for 3–5 reps for **power**, resting for 2–5 min.

2 to 3 sets for 6–8 reps for **strength**, resting for 1½–2 min.

2 to 3 sets for 8–12 reps for **growth**, resting for 1–1½ min.

2 to 3 sets for 12–20 reps for **endurance**, resting for 45 sec–1 min.

TEMPO All kettlebell movements should be performed with the intent to move quickly without compromising form or technique. **Try a tempo of 2:2 or 1:2.**

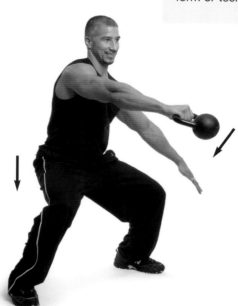

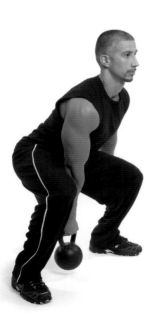

TO AVOID INJURY, DOUBLE-CHECK:

- Feet remain flat on the floor.
- Don't lock your knees.
- Back maintains its natural curve; avoid rounding your spine at any point.
- Make sure your abdominal muscles are engaged throughout the movement.
- Keep shoulders back.
- Don't flex your head forward.
- Make sure your feet aren't too close together.

kettlebell swinging snatch

This exercise takes the swing clean (see pages 72–73) one step further. Rather than having the kettlebell finishing in the rack position, it arrives overhead in the shoulder press position. The most important details are (1) the force generated and (2) the deceleration that occurs at the end phase. Grip strength is also important when slowing the kettlebell down. What makes this exercise fun is the feeling of gravity taking over, which also slows the kettlebell down. This movement is complex and will challenge your entire body.

1 Begin this movement just as if you were doing an exaggerated squat. By extending your buttocks farther back, you force a slight forward lean in your chest and torso. Firmly holding the kettlebell handle with one hand, lower your arm straight down between your legs. Remember to keep your back firm and straight.

2 Thrust your hips forward forcefully and, using the power that you generate, swing the kettlebell up, keeping your arm straight.

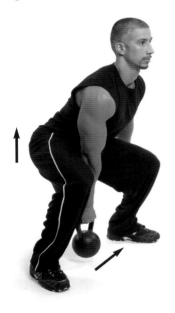

3 At this point, the momentum of the swinging force will cause you to stand up straight. Your arm and the kettlebell will swing up higher than shoulder height.

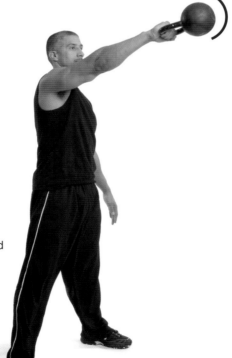

4 The initial momentum of standing will cause the kettlebell to travel over your the handle to rotate in your hand.

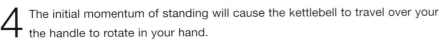

5 As this happens, lock your elbow and squat to absorb the force of the rotating kettlebell. The ending position will look like the bottom phase of an overhead rack squat position.

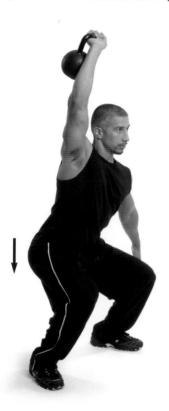

HOW MANY

2 to 3 sets for 3–5 reps for **power**, resting for 2–5 min.

2 to 3 sets for 6–8 reps for **strength**, resting for 1½–2 min.

2 to 3 sets for 8–12 reps for **growth**, resting for 1–1½ min.

2 to 3 sets for 12–20 reps for **endurance**, resting for 45 sec–1 min.

TEMPO All kettlebell movements should be performed with the intent to move quickly without compromising form or technique. **Try a tempo of 2:2 or 1:2.**

6 To return to the starting position, just reverse the path the kettlebell came up. The path the kettlebell travels in this exercise resembles a semicircle.

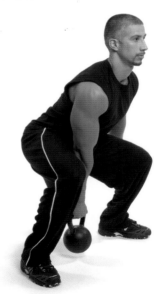

TO AVOID INJURY, DOUBLE-CHECK:

- Don't lock your knees.
- Back maintains its natural curve; avoid rounding your spine at any point.
- Make sure your abdominal muscles are engaged throughout the movement.
- Keep shoulders back.
- Don't flex your head forward.
- Make sure your feet aren't too close together.

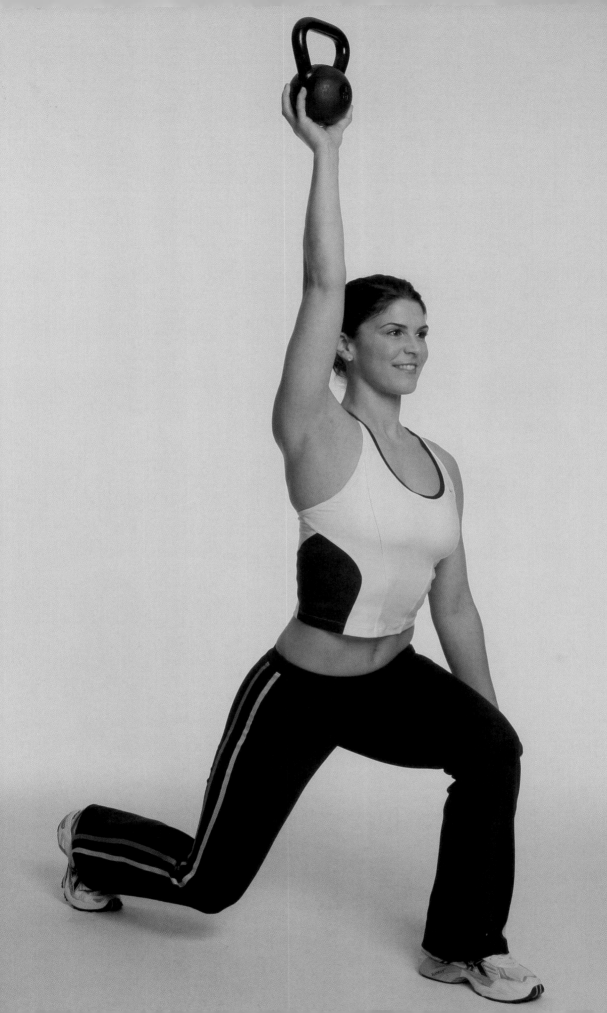

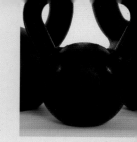

combination movements

kettlebell split squat with overhead press

Here's a way to add complexity to the split squat while working the shoulder, elbow, and wrist muscles in a dynamic way. This movement incorporates a split squat and a shoulder press at the same time. You can decide to work one or both shoulders by using the kettlebells one at a time or together.

RACK SPLIT SQUAT WITH OVERHEAD PRESS

1 Standing tall, start this movement with one foot forward and the other back. The forward foot should be flat and the back foot rising on your toes. Your arm should start in the curl position with the kettlebell resting just below your wrist. Depending on the size of the kettlebell, it may rest on your biceps.

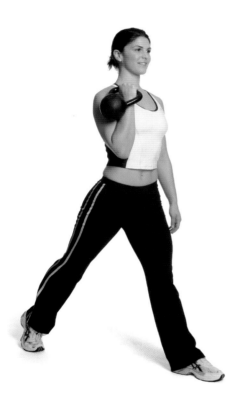

2 As your lower body descends, simultaneously push the kettlebell upward.

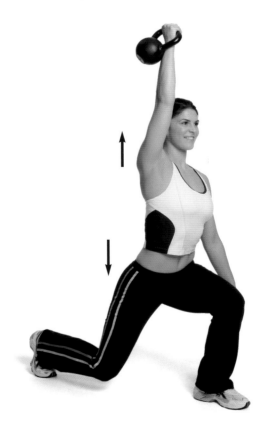

3 To return to the starting position, simultaneously push your lower body up and bring the kettlebell into the starting rack position.

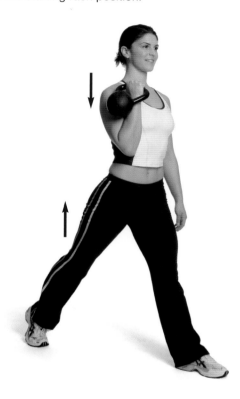

HOW MANY

2 to 3 sets for 3–5 reps for **power**, resting for 2–5 min.

2 to 3 sets for 6–8 reps for **strength**, resting for 1½–2 min.

2 to 3 sets for 8–12 reps for **growth**, resting for 1–1½ min.

2 to 3 sets for 12–20 reps for **endurance**, resting for 45 sec–1 min.

TEMPO All kettlebell movements should be performed with the intent to move quickly without compromising form or technique. **Try a tempo of 2:2 or 1:2.**

TO AVOID INJURY, DOUBLE-CHECK:

- Feet remain close enough together to retain control and balance.
- Don't lock your knees.
- Back maintains its natural curve; avoid rounding your spine at any point.
- Make sure your abdominal muscles are engaged throughout the movement.
- Keep shoulders back.
- Keep arm/elbow as close to your body as possible when the kettlebell moves upward.
- Don't flex your head forward.
- Make sure your feet aren't too close together.
- Make sure your front heel stays down.
- The kettlebell arm should be straight and close to or in line with your ear.
- Don't lean your chest too far over the front leg.

WAITER SPLIT SQUAT WITH OVERHEAD PRESS

1 Standing tall, start this movement with one foot forward and the other back. The forward foot should be flat and the back foot rising on your toes. Your arm should start in the curl position with the bottom of the kettlebell resting on your palm.

2 As your lower body descends, simultaneously push the kettlebell upward.

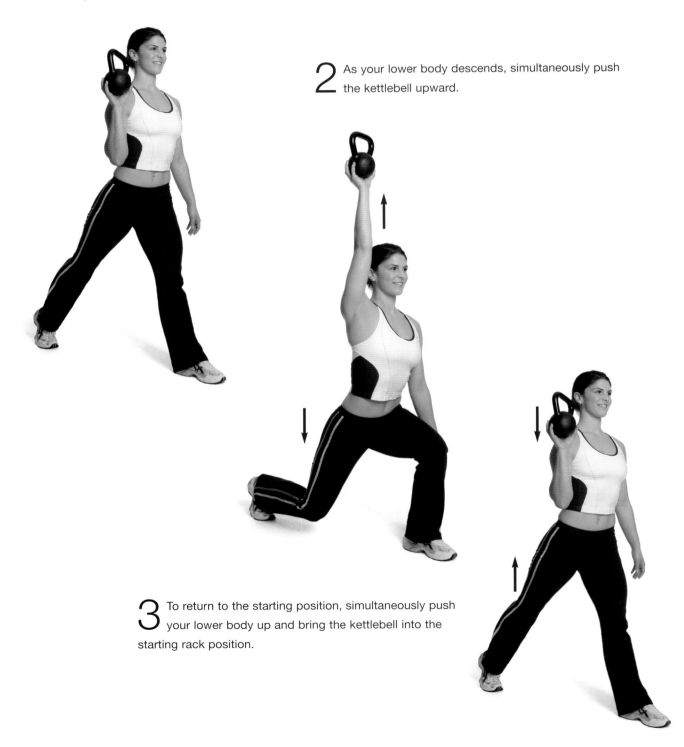

3 To return to the starting position, simultaneously push your lower body up and bring the kettlebell into the starting rack position.

BOTTOMS-UP SPLIT SQUAT WITH OVERHEAD PRESS

1 Standing tall, start this movement with one foot forward and the other back. The forward foot should be flat and the back foot rising on your toes. Your arm should start in the curl position with the handle of the kettlebell firmly in your grip and the bottom facing the ceiling.

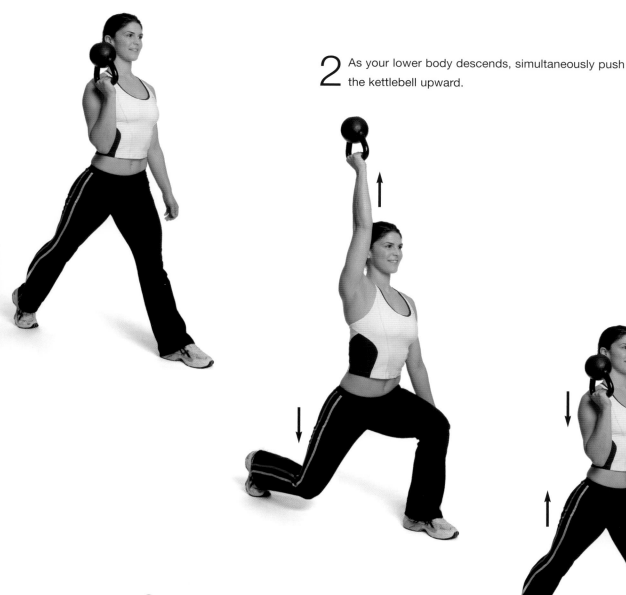

2 As your lower body descends, simultaneously push the kettlebell upward.

3 To return to the starting position, simultaneously push your lower body up and bring the kettlebell into the starting bottoms-up position.

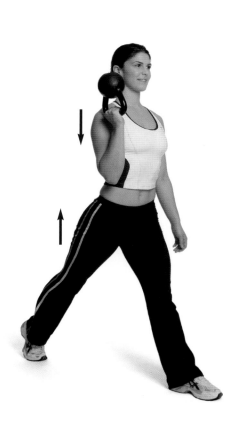

kettlebell step-back lunge with shoulder (overhead) press

The step-back lunge is another variation of the lunge. Stepping backward works on balance and weight distribution and targets all the leg muscles. This lunge challenges the stability of your front leg while stepping backward. To challenge your balance and coordination in the step-back lunge, you can add an overhead press. This will work the muscles of the shoulder while increasing the degree of difficulty of the entire exercise. You can use one or two kettlebells and vary the grip positions.

KETTLEBELL STEP–BACK LUNGE WITH RACK PRESS

1 Start this movement standing up straight with both feet together. Hold the kettlebell in the rack start position, resting it on your forearm and bicep. Keep your elbow firmly against the side of your body.

2 As you step back a comfortable distance, simultaneously begin to push the kettlebell upward. The grounded leg will be called on for support and balance.

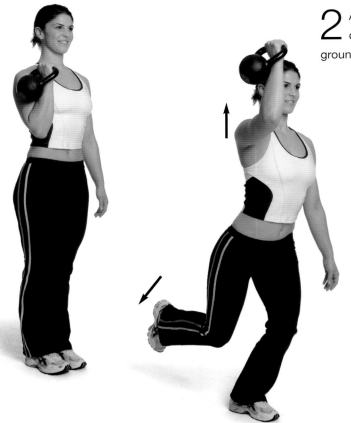

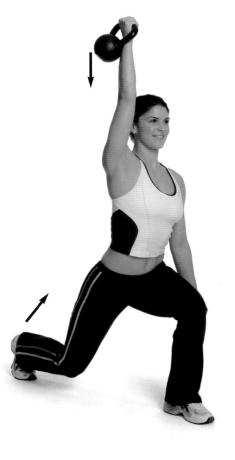

3 You'll land in the bottom or end phase of a split squat with the kettlebell over your head.

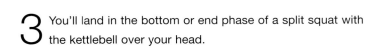

4 To return to the starting position, push your lower body up and forward and bring the kettlebell into the starting rack position.

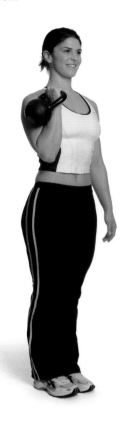

HOW MANY

2 to 3 sets for 3–5 reps for **power**, resting for 2–5 min.

2 to 3 sets for 6–8 reps for **strength**, resting for 1½–2 min.

2 to 3 sets for 8–12 reps for **growth**, resting for 1–1½ min.

2 to 3 sets for 12–20 reps for **endurance**, resting for 45 sec–1 min.

TEMPO All kettlebell movements should be performed with the intent to move quickly without compromising form or technique. **Try a tempo of 2:2 or 1:2**.

TO AVOID INJURY, DOUBLE-CHECK:

- Use the lunging foot to control distance—you should be able to maintain your balance.
- Don't lock your knees.
- Back maintains its natural curve; avoid rounding your spine at any point.
- Make sure your abdominal muscles are engaged throughout the movement.
- Keep shoulders back.
- Don't flex your head forward.
- Make sure your feet aren't too close together.
- Make sure your front heel stays down.
- The kettlebell arm should be straight and close to or in line with your ear.

KETTLEBELL STEP-BACK LUNGE WITH WAITER PRESS

1 Start this movement standing up straight with both feet together. Hold the kettlebell in the waiter position, with your elbow placed firmly against the side of your body.

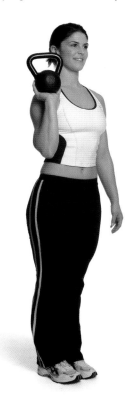

2 As you step back a comfortable distance, simultaneously begin to push the kettlebell upward. The grounded leg will be called on for support and balance.

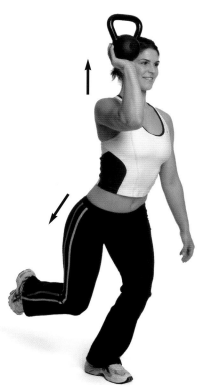

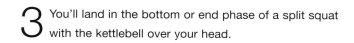

3 You'll land in the bottom or end phase of a split squat with the kettlebell over your head.

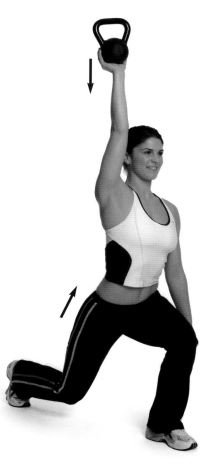

4 To return to the starting position, simultaneously push your lower body up and forward and bring the kettlebell into the starting waiter position.

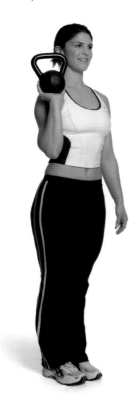

HOW MANY

2 to 3 sets for 3–5 reps for **power**, resting for 2–5 min.

2 to 3 sets for 6–8 reps for **strength**, resting for 1½–2 min.

2 to 3 sets for 8–12 reps for **growth**, resting for 1–1½ min.

2 to 3 sets for 12–20 reps for **endurance**, resting for 45 sec–1 min.

TEMPO All kettlebell movements should be performed with the intent to move quickly without compromising form or technique. **Try a tempo of 2:2 or 1:2.**

TO AVOID INJURY, DOUBLE-CHECK:

- Use the lunging foot to control distance.
- Don't lock your knees.
- Back maintains its natural curve; avoid rounding your spine at any point.
- Make sure your abdominal muscles are engaged throughout the movement.
- Keep shoulders back.
- Don't flex your head forward.
- Make sure your feet aren't too close together.
- Make sure your front heel stays down.
- The kettlebell arm should be straight and close to or in line with your ear.

KETTLEBELL STEP-BACK LUNGE WITH BOTTOMS-UP PRESS

1 Start this movement standing up straight with both feet together. The kettlebell should be in the bottoms-up position, with your elbow held firmly against the side of your body.

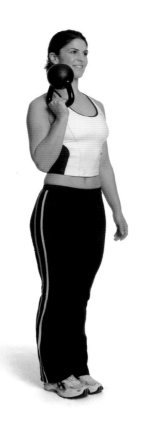

2 As you step back to a comfortable distance, simultaneously begin to push the kettlebell upward. The grounded leg will be called on for support and balance.

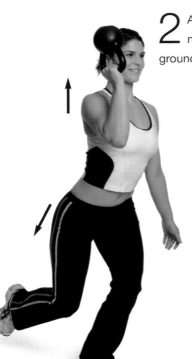

3 You'll land in the bottom or end phase of a split squat with the kettlebell over your head.

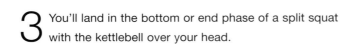
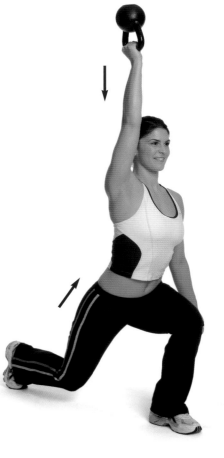

4 To return to the starting position, simultaneously push your lower body up and forward and bring the kettlebell into the starting bottoms-up position.

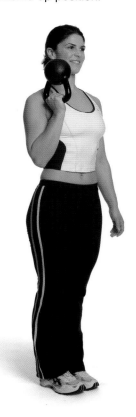

HOW MANY

2 to 3 sets for 3–5 reps for **power**, resting for 2–5 min.

2 to 3 sets for 6–8 reps for **strength**, resting for 1½–2 min.

2 to 3 sets for 8–12 reps for **growth**, resting for 1–1½ min.

2 to 3 sets for 12–20 reps for **endurance**, resting for 45 sec–1 min.

TEMPO All kettlebell movements should be performed with the intent to move quickly without compromising form or technique. **Try a tempo of 2:2 or 1:2.**

TO AVOID INJURY, DOUBLE-CHECK:

- Use the lunging foot to control distance.
- Don't lock your knees.
- Back maintains its natural curve; avoid rounding your spine at any point.
- Make sure your abdominal muscles are engaged throughout the movement.
- Keep shoulders back.
- Don't flex your head forward.
- Make sure your feet aren't too close together.
- Make sure your front heel stays down.
- The kettlebell arm should be straight and close to or in line with your ear.

kettlebell step-forward lunge with overhead press

To challenge your balance and coordination in the step forward lunge, you can add an overhead press. This will work the muscles of the shoulder while increasing the degree of difficulty of the entire exercise. You can use one or two kettlebells and vary the hand position.

STEP—FORWARD LUNGE WITH OVERHEAD PRESS (RACK)

1 Start this movement standing up straight with both feet together. With the kettlebell in the rack position, keep your elbow firmly against the side of your body.

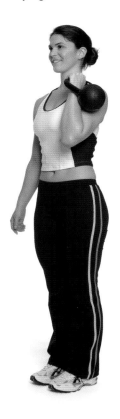

2 As you lunge forward, simultaneously begin to push the kettlebell upward. You'll land in the bottom or end phase of a split squat with the kettlebell over your head.

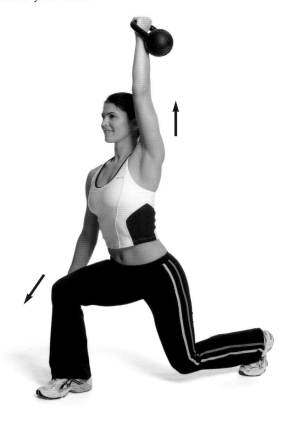

3 To return to the starting position, simultaneously push your lower body up and bring the kettlebell into the starting rack position.

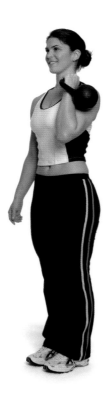

HOW MANY

2 to 3 sets for 3–5 reps for **power**, resting for 2–5 min.

2 to 3 sets for 6–8 reps for **strength**, resting for 1½–2 min.

2 to 3 sets for 8–12 reps for **growth**, resting for 1–1½ min.

2 to 3 sets for 12–20 reps for **endurance**, resting for 45 sec–1 min.

TEMPO All kettlebell movements should be performed with the intent to move quickly without compromising form or technique. **Try a tempo of 2:2 or 1:2.**

TO AVOID INJURY, DOUBLE-CHECK:

- Use the lunging foot to control distance.
- Don't lock your knees.
- Back maintains its natural curve; avoid rounding your spine at any point.
- Make sure your abdominal muscles are engaged throughout the movement.
- Keep shoulders back.
- Don't flex your head forward.
- Make sure your feet aren't too close together.
- Make sure your front heel stays down.
- The kettlebell arm should be straight and close to or in line with your ear.

STEP—FORWARD LUNGE WITH OVERHEAD PRESS (WAITER)

1 Start this movement by standing straight up with both feet together. Hold the kettlebell in the waiter position, with your elbow firmly against the side of your body.

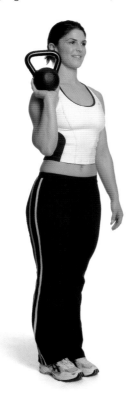

2 As you lunge forward, begin to push the kettlebell upward. You'll land in the bottom or end phase of a split squat with the kettlebell over your head.

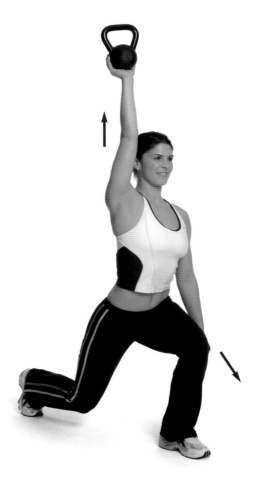

3 To return to the starting position, simultaneously push your lower body up and bring the kettlebell into the starting waiter position.

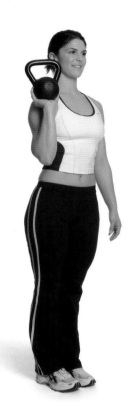

HOW MANY

2 to 3 sets for 3–5 reps for **power**, resting for 2–5 min.

2 to 3 sets for 6–8 reps for **strength**, resting for 1½–2 min.

2 to 3 sets for 8–12 reps for **growth**, resting for 1–1½ min.

2 to 3 sets for 12–20 reps for **endurance**, resting for 45 sec–1 min.

TEMPO All kettlebell movements should be performed with the intent to move quickly without compromising form or technique. **Try a tempo of 2:2 or 1:2.**

TO AVOID INJURY, DOUBLE-CHECK:

- Use the lunging foot to control distance.
- Don't lock your knees.
- Back maintains its natural curve; avoid rounding your spine at any point.
- Make sure your abdominal muscles are engaged throughout the movement.
- Keep shoulders back.
- Don't flex your head forward.
- Make sure your feet aren't too close together.
- Make sure your front heel stays down.
- The kettlebell arm should be straight and close to or in line with your ear.

STEP—FORWARD LUNGE WITH OVERHEAD PRESS (BOTTOMS—UP)

1 Start this movement by standing up straight with both feet together, with the kettlebell in the bottoms-up position and with your elbow firmly against the side of your body.

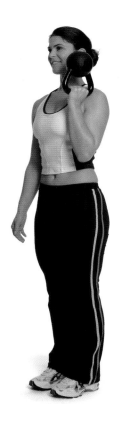

2 As you step forward, begin to push the kettlebell upward. You'll land in the bottom or end phase of a split squat with the kettlebell over your head.

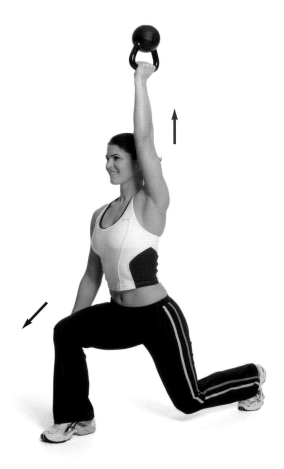

3 To return to the starting position, simultaneously push your lower body up and bring the kettlebell into the starting bottoms-up position.

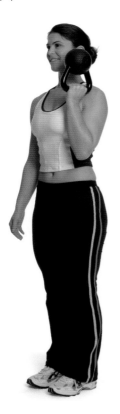

HOW MANY

2 to 3 sets for 3–5 reps for **power**, resting for 2–5 min.

2 to 3 sets for 6–8 reps for **strength**, resting for 1½–2 min.

2 to 3 sets for 8–12 reps for **growth**, resting for 1–1½ min.

2 to 3 sets for 12–20 reps for **endurance**, resting for 45 sec–1 min.

TEMPO All kettlebell movements should be performed with the intent to move quickly without compromising form or technique. **Try a tempo of 2:2 or 1:2.**

TO AVOID INJURY, DOUBLE-CHECK:

- Use the lunging foot to control distance.
- Don't lock your knees.
- Back maintains its natural curve; avoid rounding your spine at any point.
- Make sure your abdominal muscles are engaged throughout the movement.
- Keep shoulders back.
- Don't flex your head forward.
- Make sure your feet aren't too close together.
- Make sure your front heel stays down.
- The kettlebell arm should be straight and close to or in line with your ear.

kettlebell overhead squat

This is a multijoint movement focusing on total body development. This is a progression from the basic kettlebell squat illustrated on pages 16–17. This exercise strengthens every muscle in the lower body. Moving the kettlebell overhead will challenge your equilibrium and improve your abililty to stabilize a weight overhead while lowering your body into a sitting position—an excellent total-body exercise!

1 Standing with correct posture, with your feet shoulder width apart, flat on the floor, and pointed forward, hold the kettlebell overhead with one arm. You may choose one of the three grip positions for this exercise (see pages 14–15). You should start with the rack position and progress to the waiter position and then the bottoms-up position as the movement becomes easier for you and you are able to maintain control of the kettlebell overhead. Your shoulders should be pulled back and your neck elongated. You should be looking straight ahead.

2 Lower yourself as if you were going to sit on a chair. Continue to lower yourself until your hips and knees are at a ninety-degree angle. The kettlebell should remain overhead. Look at the kettlebell as you lower yourself—it will help you maintain control of the kettlebell while it is overhead. Rotate your torso slightly while squatting, and maintain a line between the arm overhead and the arm by your side.

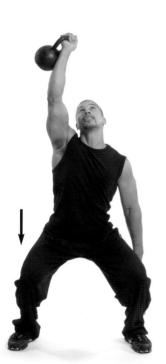

Rack

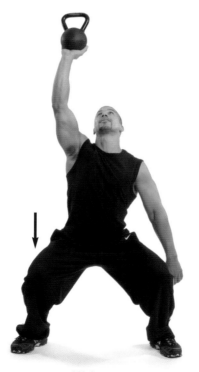

Waiter

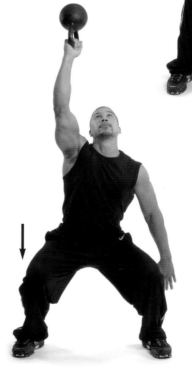

Bottoms-up

3 Return to the starting position. Be sure to check your posture before attempting another repetition.

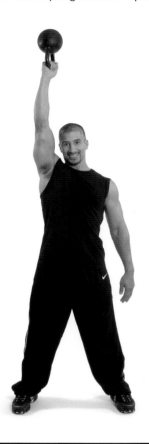

HOW MANY

2 to 3 sets for 3–5 reps for **power**, resting for 2–5 min.

2 to 3 sets for 6–8 reps for **strength**, resting for 1½–2 min.

2 to 3 sets for 8–12 reps for **growth**, resting for 1–1½ min.

2 to 3 sets for 12–20 reps for **endurance**, resting for 45 sec–1 min.

TEMPO All kettlebell movements should be performed with the intent to move quickly without compromising form or technique. **Try a tempo of 3:3.**

TO AVOID INJURY, DOUBLE-CHECK:

- Feet remain flat on the floor.
- Don't lock your knees.
- Back maintains its natural curve; avoid rounding your spine at any point.
- Make sure your abdominal muscles are engaged throughout the movement.
- Keep shoulders back.
- Don't flex your head forward.
- Remember to stop lowering yourself when your hips and knees reach a ninety-degree angle.
- If the kettlebell feels like it is going to fall while in the bottoms-up grip position, maintain a firm grip on the handle, turn your face away, and use your opposite hand to protect your face as you allow the kettlebell to fall into a racked grip position.

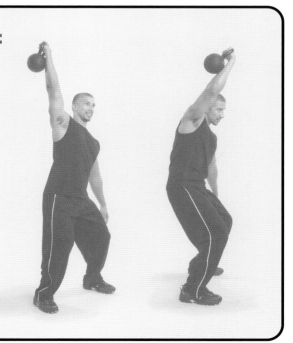

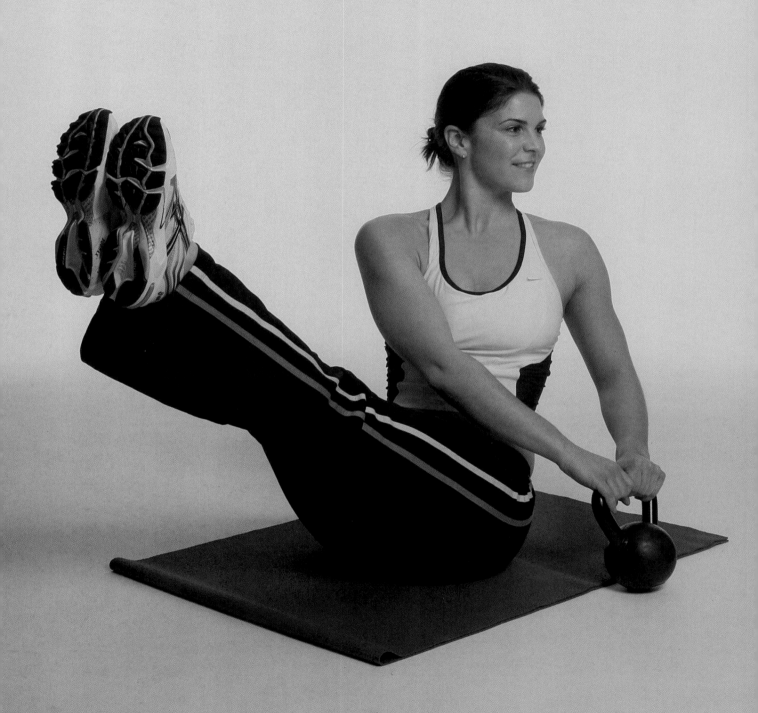

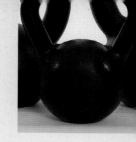

abdominal exercises

180-degree kettlebell crunch

The 180-degree crunch is a great exercise for the abdominals. Because you are holding your legs straight up, it will test your flexibility. This exercise is a weighted abdominal exercise, which will fatigue your abs much more quickly than a regular crunch.

1 While lying on your back, hold your legs straight up in the air with your heels pointing toward the ceiling. Keep your back in contact with the ground while you hold the kettlebell by its base.

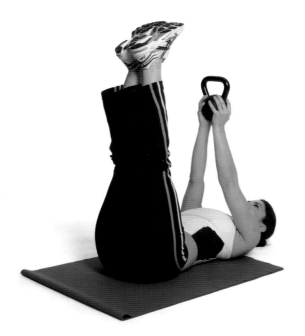

2 Try to keep your legs in a fixed position. Lift your shoulder blades off the ground toward the ceiling. This will bring your arms and the kettlebell closer to your toes.

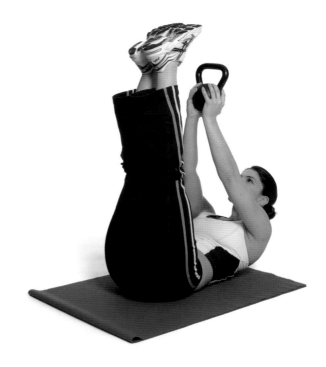

3 Keep your legs in the air, and lower your shoulders back to the ground.

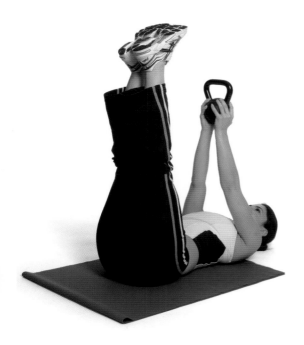

HOW MANY

2 to 3 sets for 3–5 reps for **power**, resting for 2–5 min.

2 to 3 sets for 6–8 reps for **strength**, resting for 1½–2 min.

2 to 3 sets for 8–12 reps for **growth**, resting for 1–1½ min.

2 to 3 sets for 12–20 reps for **endurance**, resting for 45 sec–1 min.

TEMPO All kettlebell movements should be performed with the intent to move quickly without compromising form or technique. **Try a tempo of 2:2 or 2:3.**

TO AVOID INJURY, DOUBLE-CHECK:

- Make sure your abdominal muscles are engaged throughout the movement.
- Keep shoulders back.
- Don't flex your head forward.
- Go up as far as your flexibility will allow without compromising form.

jackknife

Here's another weighted abdominal exercise that will strengthen your core. This exercise is difficult because each leg must meet the kettlebell in the air.

1 Lie flat on your back with arms and legs stretched out. Hold the kettlebell by its base with both hands. Keep your head on the ground with your eyes looking up.

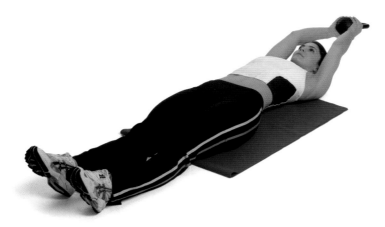

2 Simultaneously lift one leg and the kettlebell into the air to meet at the center. At this point, fix your eyes on the kettlebell. Keep the other leg straight on the ground.

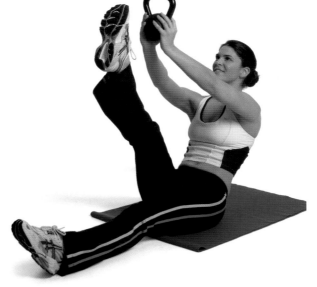

HOW MANY

2 to 3 sets for 3–5 reps for **power**, resting for 2–5 min.

2 to 3 sets for 6–8 reps for **strength**, resting for 1½–2 min.

2 to 3 sets for 8–12 reps for **growth**, resting for 1–1½ min.

2 to 3 sets for 12–20 reps for **endurance**, resting for 45 sec–1 min.

TEMPO All kettlebell movements should be performed with the intent to move quickly without compromising form or technique. **Try a tempo of 2:2 or 2:3.**

3 Simultaneously lower your leg and arms back to the starting position.

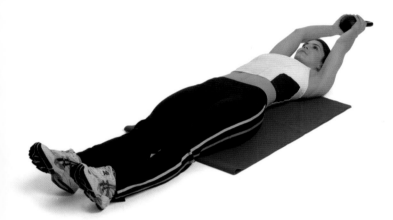

TO AVOID INJURY, DOUBLE-CHECK:

- Back maintains its natural curve; avoid rounding your spine at any point.
- Make sure your abdominal muscles are engaged throughout the movement.
- Keep shoulders back.
- Don't flex your head forward.
- Go up as far as your flexibility will allow without compromising form.

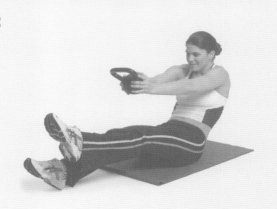

Russian twist

The Russian twist strengthens the core and the obliques while challenging your stability. The complexity of this exercise varies depending on where your feet and legs are positioned and how heavy the kettlebell is. Balance is a key component to the Russian twist, due to the twisting of the torso and the uneven loading of the kettlebell to one side of the body.

RUSSIAN TWIST (WITH STRAIGHT LEG)

In this variation of the Russian twist, your legs remain straight throughout the exercise. This brings you higher off the ground into a V position. Remember to keep your back as straight and strong as possible with your shoulders back. Try to keep your pelvis from rotating too much during the exercise.

1 Start with your feet together and raised off the ground. The distance off the ground will depend on your strength and flexibility. Hold the kettlebell by the handle with both hands. Arms are bent comfortably.

2 Rotate the kettlebell to the right side of your body. Your head and trunk should move as one with the kettlebell. Tap the kettlebell on the ground and rotate back to the middle.

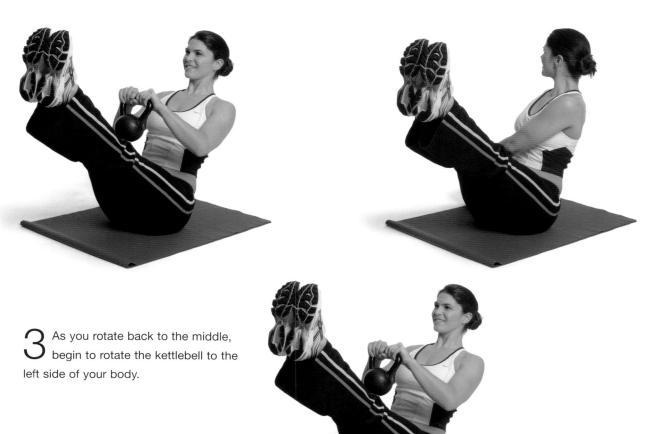

3 As you rotate back to the middle, begin to rotate the kettlebell to the left side of your body.

4 Rotate the kettlebell all the way to the left side of your body. Your head and trunk should move as one with the kettlebell. Tap the kettlebell on the ground and rotate back to the middle.

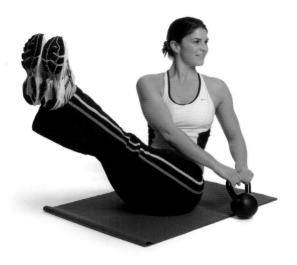

HOW MANY

2 to 3 sets for 3–5 reps for **power**, resting for 2–5 min.

2 to 3 sets for 6–8 reps for **strength**, resting for 1½–2 min.

2 to 3 sets for 8–12 reps for **growth**, resting for 1–1½ min.

2 to 3 sets for 12–20 reps for **endurance**, resting for 45 sec–1 min.

TEMPO All kettlebell movements should be performed with the intent to move quickly without compromising form or technique. **Try a tempo of 2:2 or 2:3.**

RUSSIAN TWIST (WITH BENT LEG)

Start this movement holding the kettlebell in both hands while sitting up straight. Make sure to keep your back straight, shoulders back, and your feet off the ground with knees bent at a forty-degree angle. First twist your torso to the right side and touch the kettlebell to the ground. Return to the center, then twist to the left side and tap the kettlebell on the ground.

TO AVOID INJURY, DOUBLE-CHECK:

- Back maintains its natural curve; avoid rounding your spine at any point.
- Make sure your abdominal muscles are engaged throughout the movement.
- Keep shoulders back.
- Don't flex your head forward.
- Keep kettlebell arm straight and the kettlebell facing the ceiling.
- Keep your eyes on the kettlebell at all times.
- Don't overrotate.
- Only the kettlebell should touch the ground during rotation.

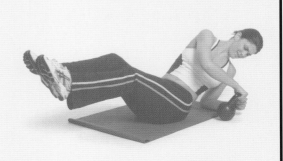

Turkish get-up rack position (with hands)

The Turkish get-up incorporates balance and strength into one challenging exercise. Because the kettle-bell stays above your head throughout the whole exercise, you end up using your entire body. Your shoulder muscles and rotator cuff are doing a lot of work because you are moving up and down while keeping the kettlebell balanced overhead. Your abdominals flex and stabilize your trunk as you are moving up and down, while your leg and hip muscles flex and stabilize your lower body.

1 Begin this exercise by lying on the ground on your back with the kettlebell in rack position in one hand. Your free hand should be on the ground to help you through the exercise because you are lifting a heavier kettlebell. Point the kettlebell directly toward the ceiling, and keep it this way throughout the entire exercise.

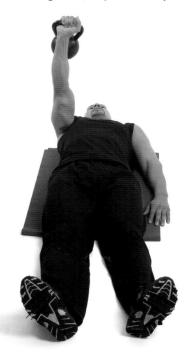

2 Use the hand on the ground to begin pushing up. Bend your right leg to transfer your weight to the kettlebell-free arm. This becomes your working arm.

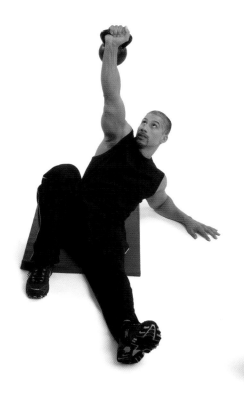

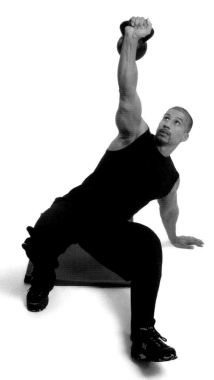

3 Use the working arm to push yourself up onto both legs, coming up higher off the ground. This exercise is different for each person because we all transfer our weight differently. Just remember to keep the kettlebell overhead and pointing straight toward the ceiling the entire time, with your eyes on it.

Come to a squat position with the kettlebell pointing up. Your legs should be shoulder width apart for added support.

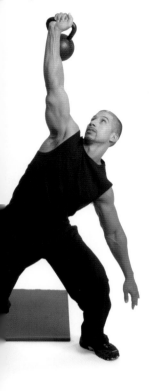

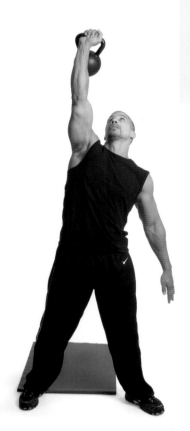

HOW MANY

2 to 3 sets for 3–5 reps for **power**, resting for 2–5 min.

2 to 3 sets for 6–8 reps for **strength**, resting for 1½–2 min.

2 to 3 sets for 8–12 reps for **growth**, resting for 1–1½ min.

2 to 3 sets for 12–20 reps for **endurance**, resting for 45 sec–1 min.

TEMPO All kettlebell movements should be performed with the intent to move quickly without compromising form or technique. **Try a tempo of 2:2 or 2:3.**

5 Stand up straight with the kettlebell perpendicular to the ceiling. Keep your feet shoulder distance apart. Begin to come back down toward the ground the same way you came up. The kettlebell should always be pointing straight toward the ceiling, and you should continue to keep your eyes on it.

6 Lower yourself to the ground the same way you came up.

TO AVOID INJURY, DOUBLE-CHECK:

- Back maintains its natural curve; avoid rounding your spine at any point.
- Make sure your abdominal muscles are engaged throughout the movement.
- Keep shoulders back.
- Don't flex your head forward.
- Keep kettlebell arm straight and the kettlebell facing the ceiling.
- Keep your eyes on the kettlebell at all times.

Turkish get-up rack position (with no hands)

The challenge in this movement is to keep the kettlebell in the air during the entire exercise. This is a great lesson in balance and adaptation. Traditionally, this exercise is performed with one kettlebell. Because the kettlebell stays above your head throughout the whole exercise, you must use your entire body to perform the exercise. The goal is to stand up and lie back down without using your hands while keeping the kettlebell overhead in the rack position. Remember to keep your eyes on the kettlebell the entire time so you do not get hit in the face.

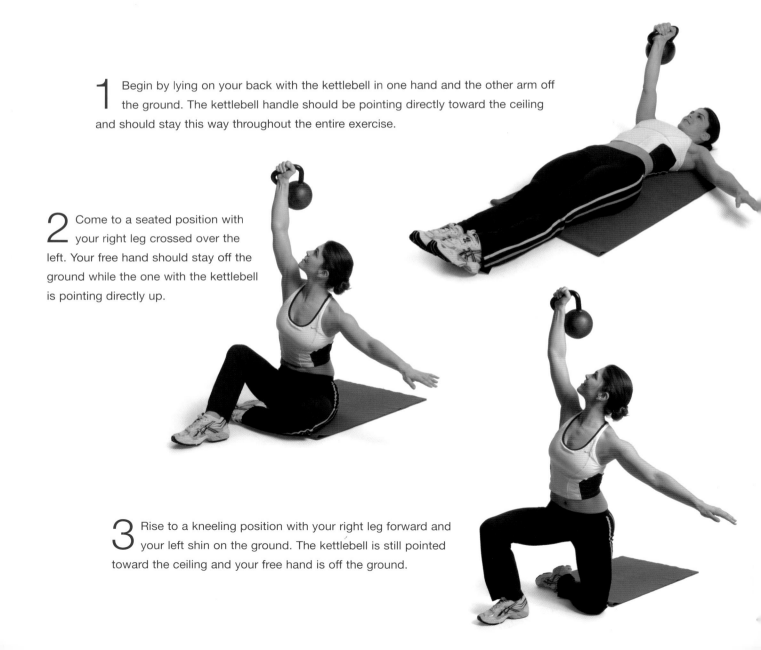

1 Begin by lying on your back with the kettlebell in one hand and the other arm off the ground. The kettlebell handle should be pointing directly toward the ceiling and should stay this way throughout the entire exercise.

2 Come to a seated position with your right leg crossed over the left. Your free hand should stay off the ground while the one with the kettlebell is pointing directly up.

3 Rise to a kneeling position with your right leg forward and your left shin on the ground. The kettlebell is still pointed toward the ceiling and your free hand is off the ground.

4 Stand onto two legs, maintaining the kettlebell overhead. Continue to keep your eyes on the kettlebell as you descend back to the starting position.

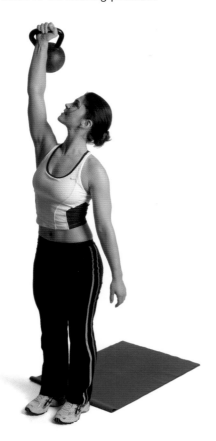

HOW MANY

2 to 3 sets for 3–5 reps for **power**, resting for 2–5 min.

2 to 3 sets for 6–8 reps for **strength**, resting for 1½–2 min.

2 to 3 sets for 8–12 reps for **growth**, resting for 1–1½ min.

2 to 3 sets for 12–20 reps for **endurance**, resting for 45 sec–1 min.

TEMPO All kettlebell movements should be performed with the intent to move quickly without compromising form or technique. **Try a tempo of 2:2 or 2:3.**

5 Lower yourself to the ground the same way you came up.

TO AVOID INJURY, DOUBLE-CHECK:

- Back maintains its natural curve; avoid rounding your spine at any point.
- Make sure your abdominal muscles are engaged throughout the movement.
- Keep shoulders back.
- Don't flex your head forward.
- Keep kettlebell arm straight and the kettlebell handle facing the ceiling.
- Keep your eyes on the kettlebell at all times.

Turkish get-up bottoms-up position (with no hands)

Like the Turkish get-up in rack position (see pages 114–115), your shoulder muscles and rotator cuff are doing a lot of work because you are moving up and down while keeping the kettlebell balanced overhead. This exercise is performed using the bottoms-up grip position. The shoulder must work much more because the kettlebell is less stable. Because of the instability, remember to begin with a lighter weight and to keep it pointing toward the ceiling the entire time.

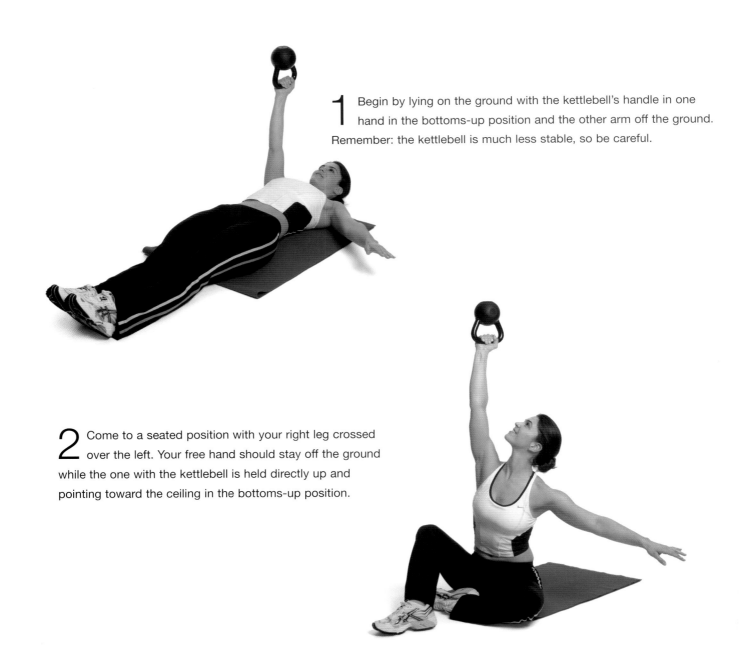

1 Begin by lying on the ground with the kettlebell's handle in one hand in the bottoms-up position and the other arm off the ground. Remember: the kettlebell is much less stable, so be careful.

2 Come to a seated position with your right leg crossed over the left. Your free hand should stay off the ground while the one with the kettlebell is held directly up and pointing toward the ceiling in the bottoms-up position.

3 Rise to a kneeling position with your right leg forward and your left shin on the ground. The kettlebell is still pointing toward the ceiling in the bottoms-up position and your free hand is off the ground.

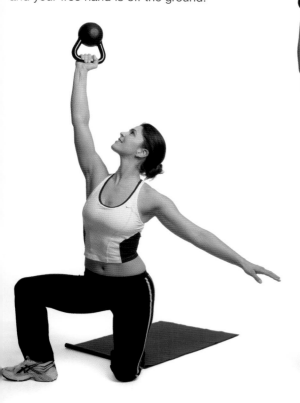

HOW MANY

2 to 3 sets for 3–5 reps for **power**, resting for 2–5 min.

2 to 3 sets for 6–8 reps for **strength**, resting for 1½–2 min.

2 to 3 sets for 8–12 reps for **growth**, resting for 1–1½ min.

2 to 3 sets for 12–20 reps for **endurance**, resting for 45 sec–1 min.

TEMPO All kettlebell movements should be performed with the intent to move quickly without compromising form or technique. **Try a tempo of 2:2 or 2:3**.

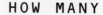

4 Stand onto both legs, maintaining the kettlebell overhead in bottoms-up position. Continue to keep your eyes on the kettlebell as you descend to the starting position, always keeping the kettlebell pointing directly up toward the ceiling.

5 Lower yourself to the ground the same way you came up.

TO AVOID INJURY, DOUBLE-CHECK:

- Back maintains its natural curve; avoid rounding your spine at any point.
- Make sure your abdominal muscles are engaged throughout the movement.
- Keep shoulders back.
- Don't flex your head forward.
- Keep kettlebell arm straight and the kettlebell facing the ceiling.
- Keep your eyes on the kettlebell at all times.

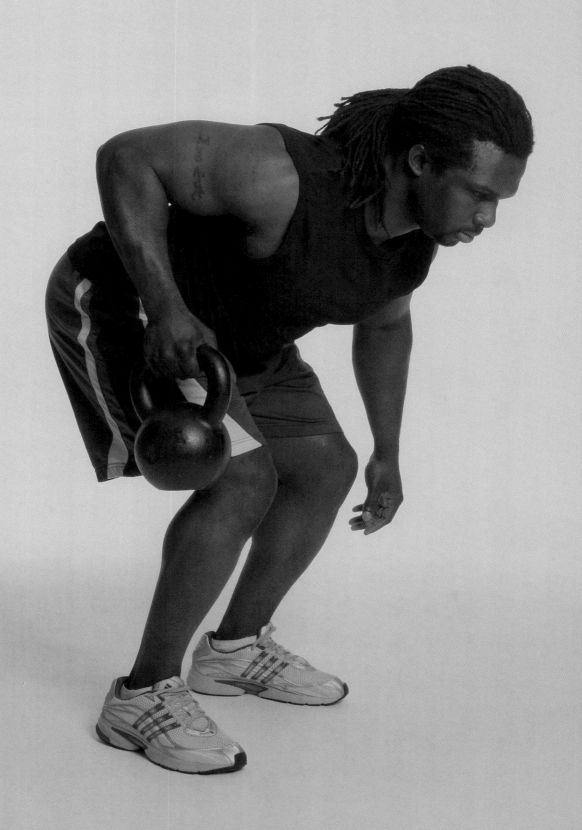

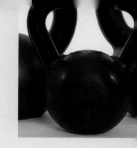

exercise routines

beginner exercise routines

Supersets are two exercises performed back to back with a rest upon completion of both exercises. The last exercise is for the abdominals.

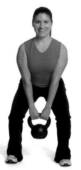

Kettlebell Squat

(pages 16–17)

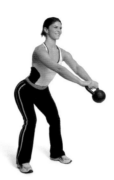

Kettlebell Double-Arm Swing Squat

(pages 20–21)

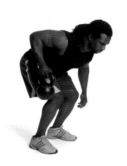

Kettlebell Bent-Over Row

(pages 36–37)

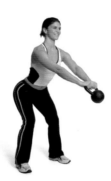

Kettlebell Double-Arm Swing Squat

(pages 20–21)

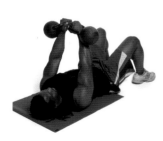

Kettlebell Chest Press

(pages 30–31)

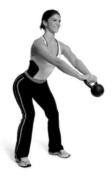

Kettlebell Double-Arm Swing Squat

(pages 20–21)

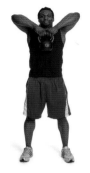

Kettlebell Upright Row

(pages 46–47)

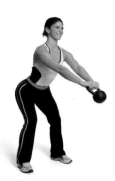

Kettlebell Double-Arm Swing Squat

(pages 20–21)

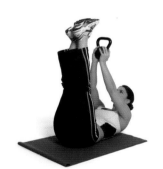

180-Degree Kettlebell Crunch

(pages 106–107)

intermediate exercise routines

Supersets are two exercises performed back to back with a rest upon completion of both exercises. The last exercise is for the abdominals.

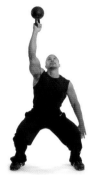

Kettlebell Overhead Squat

(pages 102–103)

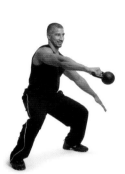

Kettlebell Single-Arm Swing Squat

(pages 68–69)

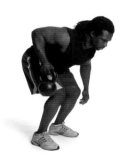

Kettlebell Bent-Over Row

(pages 36–37)

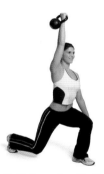

Kettlebell Split Squat with Overhead Press

(pages 86–87)

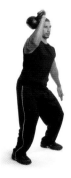

Kettlebell Swing Clean with Push Press

(pages 74–77)

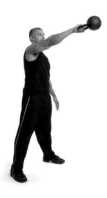

Kettlebell Swing Clean

(pages 72–73)

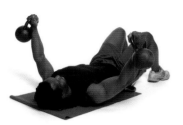

Kettlebell Chest Fly

(pages 34–35)

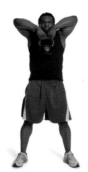

Kettlebell Double-Arm High Pull

(pages 60–61)

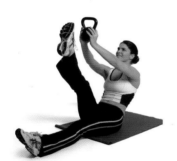

Jackknife

(pages 108–109)

advanced exercise routines

Supersets are two exercises performed back to back with a rest upon completion of both exercises. The last two exercises are for the abdominals.

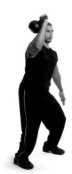

Kettlebell Push Press

(pages 64–65)

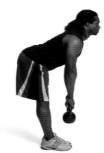

Kettlebell Stiff-Leg Dead Lift

(pages 28–29)

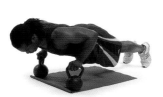

Kettlebell Push-Ups

(pages 32–33)

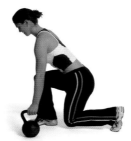

Kettlebell Step-Forward Pickups

(pages 56–57)

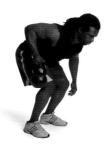

Kettlebell Bent-Over Row

(pages 36–37)

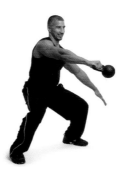

Kettlebell Alternating Swing Squat

(pages 70–71)

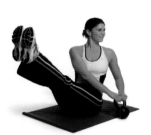

Russian Twist

(pages 110–111)

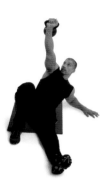

Turkish Get-Up Rack Position (with hands)

(pages 112–113)

conclusion

At this point, you should have made it through your beginner, intermediate, and advanced kettlebell exercise programs. You have no doubt noticed changes in your entire body if you have been diligently following your kettlebell program. As stated in the beginning of the book, kettlebells are excellent for anyone wanting to increase lean muscle mass, lose weight, and get the most efficient full-body workout.

Our goal for this book was to offer you a good basis and understanding of what kettlebells can offer you. To pursue kettlebells even further, we suggest referring to our list of online resources and obtaining additional educational materials. Also, if you would like to continue to learn and progress to more advanced movements, I suggest getting a certified kettlebell instructor to help train you.

resources

EQUIPMENT

Here are some useful Web sites if you would like to have your very own kettlebell.

www.power-systems.com

www.russiankettlebells.com

www.uskettlebells.com

INSTRUCTOR TRAINING

Kettlebell Concept's CEC/U–approved Instructor Training is structured in an evolving, multitiered format.

www.kettlebellconcepts.com

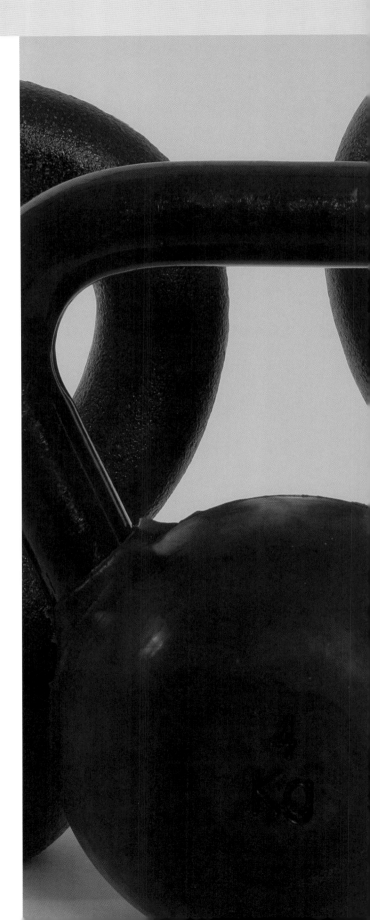

index

acknowledgments

I would like to thank my family: father and mother, Michael and Michelle Vatel, and the sensational six—Adrian Bailey, Bruce Prescod, Johnnie Godette, Trevon Jason, St. Patrick Reid, and myself, for supporting one another through so many years. Thank you to my kettlebell students Paul Winston and Gabrielle Schooley for not being afraid of something new and for all their hard work. Thanks to the Gray bar trainers for being the best at what they do. Special appreciation and thanks go to Jessica Ingraham and Raphael Garcia for modeling in this book and to Liz Minton for introducing me to kettlebells. Julie and Abby, thank you for giving Victoria and me the chance to write this book. And lastly, thank you Victoria for working with me.

—Smith Vatel, BS, CSCS

I would like to thank Julie Trelstad for recognizing talent and giving us the opportunity to write this book. I would like to extend a very special thank-you to my personal support system: Damian Mays, Paola Martinetti, and Cindy Vanlooy, who kept me going even when I felt like there wasn't enough time. I am extremely grateful to have a coauthor, Smith Vatel, and editor, Abby Rabinowitz, who understood what it took to complete a project. A great big thank-you goes to all my friends, clients, and the Wall Street Equinox trainers who stood by and supported me even though it seemed that I had too much on my plate. Finally, all of this could not have been accomplished were it not for my supportive family, who always told me that the sky's the limit.

—Victoria D. Gray, MPA, ATC

$12.95
Can. $18.95

Achieve maximum fitness using a minimum of equipment with a kettlebells workout.

Russian strongmen and weight-lifting enthusiasts have always known *the secret* to a strong, lean, powerful, and flexible body lies in a kettlebells workout.

Kettlebells, weights that look like bowling balls with a handle, have been used for years by the military and athletes.

Now you can use them to maintain and develop increased strength and fitness. Unlike dumbbells and barbells, lifted kettlebells can be used both as simple weights or swung as a pendulum—a movement that will help you develop both explosive power and agile grace.

Kettlebells provide a quick way to:

- **Lose fat**
- **Gain cardiovascular endurance**
- **Increase flexibility**
- **Develop lean muscle mass**
- **Improve sports performance and martial arts ability**

Written by certified trainers, *Kettlebells* includes a variety of exercises and sample routines so that you can work out at home or the gym—wherever it is convenient for you.

For more information, go to www.kettlebellconcepts.com/book

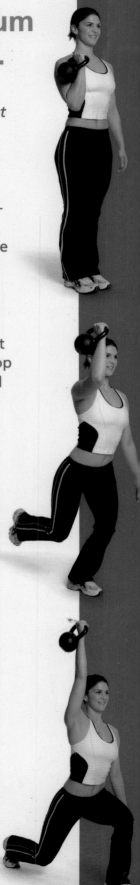

ISBN-13: 978-1-4027-2758-0
ISBN-10: 1-4027-2758-5

5 1295>

9 781402 727580

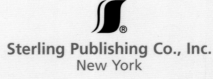

Sterling Publishing Co., Inc.
New York

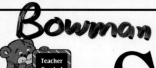

TCM 251

THEMATIC UNIT
SEASONS

Reproducible

Early Childhood

• **Literature-Based**

• **Across the Curriculum**

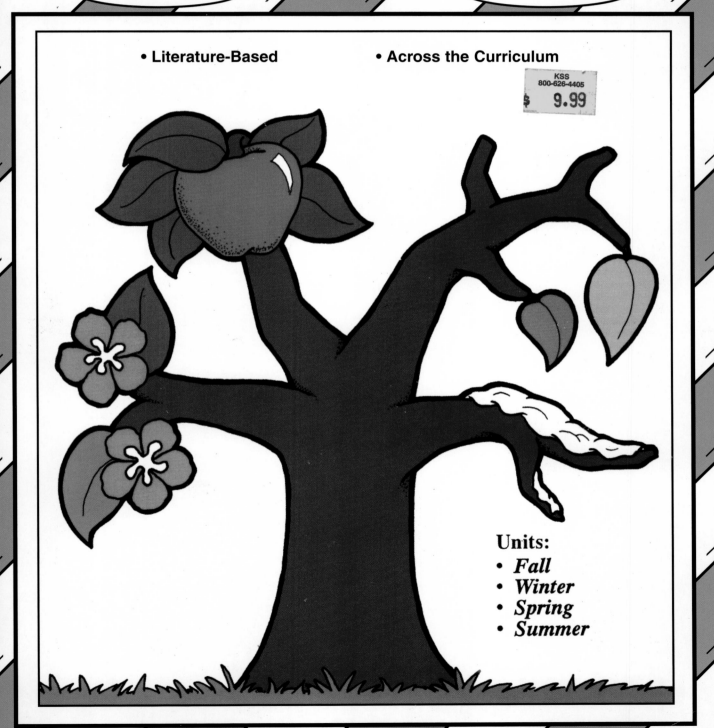

Units:
• *Fall*
• *Winter*
• *Spring*
• *Summer*

Teacher Created Materials, Inc.

Bowman
Thematic Units

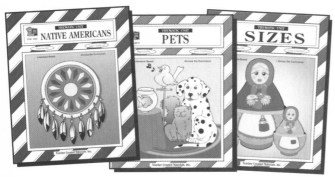

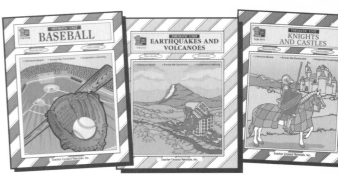

Early Childhood

TCM2614—Alphabet
TCM0250—Animals
TCM2620—Bugs
TCM2616—Colors
TCM0253—Community Workers
TCM2110—Families
TCM2059—Farm
TCM2373—Food and Nutrition
TCM0584—My Body
TCM2469—My Home and My Neighborhood
TCM0252—My World

TCM2581—Native Americans
TCM2617—Numbers
TCM2619—Pets
TCM0244—Plants
TCM0255—Safety
TCM0254—Sea Animals
TCM0251—Seasons
TCM2615—Shapes
TCM2582—Sizes
TCM2111—Things That Go
TCM2612—Weather

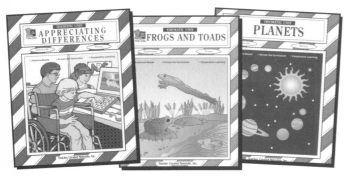

Primary

TCM2113—Ants
TCM0266—Apples
TCM2369—Appreciating Differences
TCM2376—Bats
TCM0267—Bears
TCM0256—Birds
TCM0264—Birthdays
TCM2372—Butterflies
TCM2118—Chocolate
TCM0259—Christmas
TCM2379—Clothing
TCM0279—Color
TCM0268—Creepy Crawlies
TCM0271—Dragons & Dinosaurs
TCM0261—Easter & St. Patrick's Day
TCM0246—Fairy Tales
TCM0270—Five Senses
TCM0278—Food
TCM0274—Friendship
TCM3086—Frogs and Toads
TCM3101—Gingerbread
TCM2112—Grandparents
TCM0257—Halloween
TCM2117—Ice Cream
TCM2367—Kites

TCM2370—Ladybugs
TCM2377—Magnets
TCM2365—Mice
TCM0586—My Country
TCM0276—Native Americans
TCM0272—Our Environment
TCM2375—Owls
TCM2374—Pasta and Pizza
TCM0248—Peace
TCM0277—Penguins
TCM3076—Planets
TCM0263—Popcorn
TCM0262—Presidents' Day & Martin Luther King, Jr. Day
TCM2116—Quilts
TCM2114—Rivers and Ponds
TCM0265—Rocks & Soil
TCM0269—Self-Esteem
TCM2371—Silkworms and Mealworms
TCM2580—Telling Time
TCM0258—Thanksgiving
TCM0249—Tide Pools & Coral Reefs
TCM0260—Valentine's Day
TCM0273—Weather

Intermediate

TCM2378—Amphibians and Reptiles
TCM3102—Baseball
TCM0239—Chocolate
TCM0593—Cowboys
TCM0238—Dinosaurs
TCM2591—Earthquakes and Volcanoes
TCM0286—Ecology
TCM0236—Electricity
TCM0281—Flight
TCM0280—Friends
TCM0240—Geology
TCM0241—Gold Rush
TCM0235—The Human Body
TCM0589—Ice Cream
TCM0234—Immigration

TCM0592—Insects
TCM0232—Inventions
TCM0283—Jungle
TCM2774—Knights & Castles
TCM0237—Money
TCM0230—Multicultural Folk Tales
TCM0285—Native Americans
TCM0284—Oceans
TCM0233—Peace
TCM0460—Quilts
TCM0587—Space
TCM0591—Spiders
TCM0588—Sports
TCM0242—Tall Tales
TCM0231—Water
TCM0282—Westward Ho

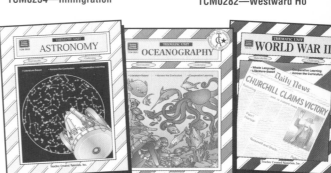

Challenging

TCM0590—African Americans
TCM0578—Ancient China
TCM0292—Ancient Egypt
TCM0297—Ancient Greece
TCM0577—Ancient India
TCM0579—Ancient Japan
TCM0573—Ancient Middle East
TCM0596—Ancient Rome
TCM0296—Archaeology
TCM2622—Astronomy
TCM0461—Chocolate
TCM0290—Civil War
TCM0597—Colonial America
TCM2364—The Depression
TCM0288—Explorers

TCM0210—Holocaust
TCM0294—Industrial Revolution
TCM0595—Mayans, Aztecs & Incas
TCM0291—Medieval Times
TCM2621—Oceanography
TCM2060—Our Legal System
TCM0580—Renaissance
TCM0293—Revolutionary War
TCM2613—Slavery
TCM0295—Transcontinental Railroad
TCM0582—U.S. Constitution
TCM0599—Vietnam War
TCM0583—Wolves
TCM0598—World War I
TCM0581—World War II

Oceanography has received the *Learning®* Magazine 2001 Teachers' Choice Award℠

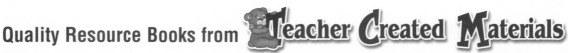

Quality Resource Books from Teacher Created Materials